THE MAMABAKE BOOK

THE MAMA BAKE BOOK

MICHELLE SHEARER
& KAREN SWAN

ABC
Books

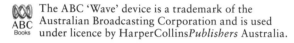 The ABC 'Wave' device is a trademark of the Australian Broadcasting Corporation and is used under licence by HarperCollins*Publishers* Australia.

First published in Australia in 2016
by HarperCollins*Publishers* Australia Pty Limited
ABN 36 009 913 517
harpercollins.com.au

HarperCollins*Publishers*
Level 13, 201 Elizabeth Street, Sydney, NSW 2000, Australia
Unit D1, 63 Apollo Drive, Rosedale, Auckland 0632, New Zealand
A 53, Sector 57, Noida, UP, India
1 London Bridge Street, London, SE1 9GF, United Kingdom
2 Bloor Street East, 20th floor, Toronto, Ontario M4W 1A8, Canada
195 Broadway, New York, NY 10007

National Library of Australia Cataloguing-in-Publication data:

Shearer, Michelle, author.
  The MamaBake book / Michelle Shearer & Karen Swan.
  ISBN: 978 0 7333 3529 7 (paperback)
  ISBN: 978 1 4607 0704 3 (ebook)
  Includes index.
  Cooking.
  Quick and easy cooking.
  Other Creators/Contributors:
  Swan, Karen, author.
  MamaBake (Australia)
641.5

Cover and internal design by Hazel Lam, HarperCollins Design Studio
Typeset in Sabon LT Std by Kirby Jones
Printed and bound in Australia by Griffin Press
The papers used by HarperCollins in the manufacture of this book are natural, recyclable product made from wood grown in sustainable plantation forests. The fibre source and manufacturing processes meet recognised international environmental standards, and carry certification.

Michelle
For my Grandmother, Doris Bird.

Karen
For my Father, Ken Swan.

CONTENTS

Part 2: Big Batch Recipes 364

The MamaBake Story

MamaBake began in April 2010, after the birth of my second child, Alby. One afternoon when picking up my older daughter, Mia, from school, I was greeted by a close friend, Bec, bearing an Esky. In that Esky was a huge family-sized lasagne for dinner that night. I took the lasagne home and realised dinner for that evening was done. I didn't have to think about it; I didn't have to pull something together! I went surfing instead of rushing around trying to get food on the table.

I wanted to reciprocate Bec's kind gesture, which got me thinking about how hard it can be sometimes as a mother to receive assistance, kindness and help from others. I felt like I needed to give back to Bec, which is natural; but I wanted all mums to experience the freedom that comes from not having to think about, prepare, cook and clear away dinner every night and wondered how that might happen in today's frantic world. And, so, I came up with MamaBake – a baking community where mothers get together in their local neighbourhood to cook one big batch meal each and then share the dish with the others, resulting in everyone going home with a week's worth of freshly cooked, homemade dinners. No funky feelings about receiving something – just a lovely, big group cook-up, where everyone pitches in and swaps their wares. Simple!

The first-ever MamaBake group started in Lennox Head, NSW, with me, Naomi, Jodie and Bec. We each went home with Chicken Stew, Chilli Con Carne, Sushi, homemade rye bread rolls and soup. It was a brilliant result and so easy. The following week, the group doubled and eventually grew so large that we eventually had to divide ourselves up.

Soon after, Karen Swan, a devout MamaBaker based in Canberra, took her newfound passion to another level and joined me to run the ever-growing MamaBake movement.

MamaBake went online in May 2010, and numbers went up and up as more women tuned in to the concept. The media soon discovered us, and MamaBake groups started springing up across Australia, Europe and the United States.

Free time and community aside, the other benefit from the MamaBake baking sessions was that the kids all got to spend time together, as well as getting involved in the food prep and cooking. New, lasting friendships were formed, experiences and woes were shared and eased – sharing the cooking turned into sharing childcare, helping with house moves, gardening, laundry.

Together, we created a beautiful, tightknit community around sharing our daily work, which significantly lightened our load, and connected us strongly to other mothers in our neighbourhoods.

– Michelle

An Introduction to MamaBake

MamaBake is all about you, the Mum (or Dad!): you're at the helm of the family, you think about what's for dinner, what's going in the lunchboxes, why that sandwich didn't get eaten, what you're cooking next week so you know what to shop for. Along with all the other responsibilities that come with motherhood, feeding our families is relentless.

And of course, as with all families, there are times when we are exhausted, uninspired and plain old just don't feel like cooking. Except, often there is no alternative to providing the family meal. Well, not always, but let's be honest, it happens a lot of the time!

And so, enter MamaBake stage left.

MamaBake, at its very core, is about mothers getting together to bake big batch meals to share out, so everyone has freshly cooked, homemade dinners ready to go for the week ahead.

MamaBake groups bring mothers together in our local neighbourhoods. Working side by side, up to our necks in egg and flour, we cook up big batch meals while the kids play around us and help prepare the ingredients. Once the meals are cooked, family-sized meals are shared out and we go home to fill the fridge or freezer.

However, our busy lifestyles and circumstances might mean that it's not possible to gather a group of mums and their children to cook together for a few hours. This book acknowledges our different situations and subsequently is designed not only for the individual MamaBaker but also for members of an active MamaBake group.

Once-A-Week Cooking Plans

If you are a solo MamaBaker, the Once-A-Week Cooking Plans have been created with you in mind. Each themed plan provides not only step-by-step preparation and cooking instructions but also a detailed shopping list so you don't have to think about anything except on which day of the week you're going to serve the meals.

Big Batch Recipes

The single Big Batch Recipes are perfect for when meat or a similar ingredient is on special, so that you can cook up a big batch meal and either share it at a MamaBake session, or simply stash it away in your freezer for a rainy day.

We all know the dreaded witching hour at the end of the day: the kids are going ballistic and we are done. There is no better feeling in the world than knowing that you have back-up in the form of a homemade, delicious family meal in the freezer, ready to go.

And here's the wrap with MamaBake: when you get together with others you're not just going home with a box full of homemade meals for your family and a week off from cooking, you're going home full of smiles, shared experiences and knowing that we are all truly in this together.

MamaBake Storage & Reheating Guide

Storage

Does your freezer look like mine used to? Enough ice coating the sides and top to give you the impression you've just opened the door to an Antarctic ice cave? Random bags and containers with barely recognisable solid lumps of something or other, stashed away because really, you had no idea what to do with it? Quite frankly, there have been years in my life when the only recognisable consumable in my freezer was a bottle of vodka and a tray of ice cubes!

As tempting as grabbing that bottle of vodka may be in the early, hazy days of motherhood, what we need from our freezers is a well organised, well-labelled bounty of homemade meals that require little-to-no effort on our part other than to defrost and reheat.

On those evenings when your baby is seemingly attached to you with Velcro, your other children are running amok and you're delirious with sleep deprivation, a well-stocked freezer the MamaBake way will be a lifeboat on the stormy seas of Motherhood.

Whether you decide to refrigerate or freeze the meal will depend on when your family will be eating it. There are refrigeration and freezing instructions with each recipe. Generally speaking most meals can be kept in the fridge for around two days.

Freezer Timeline

Soups	4 months
Savoury & sweet pies with pastry crust	4 months
Stews & casseroles (meat, chicken, vegetable)	3 months
Baked goods (cakes, etc.)	3 months
Meals containing seafood	1 month

Thawing & Reheating

This can be the biggest hurdle when it comes to frozen meals: how to safely defrost and reheat food without fear of poisoning your entire family. To reheat safely, whether you use a microwave, oven, or stovetop, it's vital to ensure that the food is thoroughly defrosted and heated through evenly. Don't rush the reheating process! There's nothing worse, and potentially dangerous, than a dish that is steaming hot on the edges, and cold and gluggy in the middle.

Defrosting Tips

1. Meat, poultry and fish (and meals containing them) need to be defrosted overnight in the fridge to avoid any bacteria forming.
2. Bakery items like cakes can be thawed at room temperature.

Containers & Labelling

I used to have one night a week that I called, 'Freezer Surprise!' night, where I would remove a container of what I thought might have been soup, but was most likely Bolognese sauce, from the depths of my freezer, and that would be dinner!

These days, I am more organised and have learned that a clearly labelled container or zip lock bag listing what's inside removes any unfortunate guesswork. Labelling the date on the container also ensures that once defrosted and reheated, your food will retain its texture and taste because it won't have been 'over-frozen' and therefore inedible.

The right container or wrapping can make or break the freezing process. Badly stored freezer food will likely dry out, burn and get covered in teeny icicles. Fine if you're an ice block on a stick, but not so great if you're a sausage! Spend a little time making sure your food is correctly stored to avoid disappointing taste and textures on reheating.

Part 1:
Once-A-Week
Cooking Plans

Once-A-Week Cooking Plans

These plans are designed to free you up from thinking and making dinners for an entire week. The aim is that you only cook once a week for 3–5 hours, and have a week's worth of family meals to store away and pull out when you're ready to serve them. We've created some guidelines to help you before you dive headlong into this brave new world of free time!

1. Prepare a shopping list: scan your pantry, fridge and freezer for ingredients you might already have.

2. Go shopping: the plans include a list with all the required ingredients so you don't have to think about it.

3. Clear your fridge and freezer as much as possible, so there is enough space for a week's worth of meals.

4. Clear your kitchen bench space – you're going to need it.

5. If you would prefer to cook alone, set the kids up with an activity – a great movie or spending time with Nana!

6. Prepare the ingredients: all of our plans detail each preparation step, so you can relax knowing that we have done the thinking for you.

7. Cook each meal according to the plan.

8. Clear up as you go so the end pots and pans aren't too intimidating.

9. Allow all meals to cool completely before storing.

10. The only thing then left to do is to decide which meal to serve on which day of the week – trust us, there's no feeling like it in the world!

MamaBake Mums have reviewed our plans and one mum, Sally, offers up these tips to any Mum about to embark on their first Once-A-Week Cooking adventure:

1. Make space on your kitchen bench and in your fridge and freezer.

2. Think ahead about what pots and pans you're going to need.

3. Don't buy ingredients for serving unless they will keep well (e.g. taco shells or pasta), or you're planning on eating the meals that week.

The 'I Don't Have Time to Cook' Plan

The 'I Don't Have Time to Cook' Plan

We get it – you want to prepare home-cooked food for your family; you know it's cheaper and better for everyone but you just don't know where to start or you just don't have the time! One of our favourite internet memes of all time is a picture of someone saying, "I read recipes like I read science fiction: I get to the end and say 'Well, that's not going to happen.'"

Yes, we know that feeling all too well and that's why these recipes are for you, dear MamaBaker who does not like cooking that much. This plan is designed juuust for you!

MamaBaker Emma says about this plan:

"These are some of the first meals I learned to cook as a young adult. There is limited need to cut onions or garlic here, but a few recipes do need a little chopping.

"You can either cook these meals quickly on the stove, or throw the ingredients together and bake or simmer and pretty much forget about them."

MamaBaker Theresa's top tips:

1. Set yourself a timer on your phone to prevent burnt meals.
2. Use shortcuts such as already-seasoned and flavoured sausage meat.
3. Choose cuts of meat and fish that don't require much cutting or boning, if any.
4. Use spices to kick up the flavour with little effort. Spices can also be used to add flavour instead of caramelising vegetables or meat.

Menu

Easiest Ever Meatloaf

Smoked Salmon Fishcakes

Wiener Schnitzel

Beef Tacos

Sausage & Mushroom 'Bolognese'

Easy Lentil Soup

One-Pan Chicken

Shopping List

Meat & Fish	Fruit & Veg	Dairy & Frozen
800 g beef mince	2 onions	100 g butter
800 g pork loin, deboned	1 red onion	1 cup milk
300 g pork mince	1 garlic bulb	5 eggs
600 g good quality pork sausages	3 carrots	200 g mozzarella
500 g chicken drumsticks	9 large potatoes	
240 g chicken thighs, boneless	2 red capsicums	
400 g smoked salmon	12 button mushrooms	
	7 handfuls baby spinach	
	1 bunch thyme	
	1 bunch rosemary	
	1 bunch coriander	
	1 bunch oregano	
	1 bunch dill	
	1 bunch chives	
	1 bunch parsley	
	3 lemons	
	1 lime	
	½ iceberg lettuce	
	4 tomatoes	
	1 avocado	

Tins, Jars & Dry Goods	Pantry Essentials	Other Ingredients
1 x 400 g tin whole peeled tomatoes	canola, sunflower or grapeseed oil	100 ml red wine
1 x 700 ml jar tomato passata	olive oil	12 taco shells or soft flour tortillas
1 cup green lentils	200 g flour	Tabasco sauce (optional)
590 g breadcrumbs	1 litre vegetable stock	
	1 tbs tomato paste	
	2 tsp brown sugar	
	salt	
	pepper	
	2 tbs mustard	
	100 ml tomato sauce (ketchup)	
	½ tsp chilli powder	
	1 tsp ground coriander	
	7 tsp ground cumin	
	2 tsp garlic powder	
	2 tsp sweet paprika	

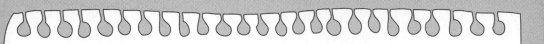

Serving Size

Each meal serves a family of 4 (approximately)

Preparation time

3 hours

Equipment

Preparation: sharp knives, chopping boards suitable for vegetables and fruit, meat and fish, kitchen scales, measuring cups and spoons, vegetable peeler, grater, citrus zester, potato masher, mixing bowls in assorted sizes, rolling pin, whisk, mixing spoons, plastic wrap, paper towel.

Cooking: large, heavy-based frying pan, medium-sized and large saucepans, loaf tin, deep baking dish (disposable aluminium baking dishes are also handy when bulk cooking).

Storage: zip lock bags, airtight containers suitable for freezing, foil.

Storage & Reheating

All of these meals are freezer-friendly and can be frozen for 1–3 months. Some need to be defrosted overnight, while other items can be baked from frozen. Most dishes will also last from several days to a week in the fridge, but we would only recommend keeping meals in the fridge if you know the order in which you plan to eat them.

Once-A-Week Cooking Preparation

	Total	Easiest Ever Meatloaf	Smoked Salmon Fishcakes	Wiener Schnitzel
Fresh Produce				
Onions	2	1 finely chopped		
Red Onion	1			
Garlic heads	2			
Carrots	3	1 grated		
Potatoes	9		5 peeled	
Capsicum	2			
Mushrooms	12			
Baby spinach leaves (handfuls)	7			
Thyme	1			
Rosemary	1			
Oregano	1			
Dill	1		1 bunch, leaves finely chopped	
Chives	1		1 bunch, finely chopped	
Parsley	1			
Lemon	3		1 zested	1 cut into wedges
Lime	1			
Meat & Fish				
Beef mince	800 g	reserve 300 g		
Pork mince	300 g	300 g		
Pork loin	800 g			deboned, cut into 6 pieces
Pork sausages	600 g			
Smoked salmon	400 g		roughly chopped	

Beef Tacos	Sausage & Mushroom 'Bolognese'	Easy Lentil Soup	One-Pan Chicken
		1 finely chopped	
			1 cut into 8 chunks
		4 cloves, finely chopped	8 cloves, peeled and bashed
		2 finely diced	
			4 cut into 8 chunks
			2 red, deseeded and cut into 10 pieces
	12 thinly sliced		
	reserve 3 handfuls	reserve 4 handfuls	
		4 sprigs, leaves picked	6 sprigs, leaves picked
			6 sprigs, leaves picked
1 bunch, leaves picked (Beef Tacos)			
			1 bunch, leaves chopped
		1 juiced	
1 juiced			
reserve 500 g			
	casings removed		

Once-A-Week Cooking Plan

1. Preheat the oven to 180°C.

2. Mix and form the **Easiest Ever Meatloaf** and bake for
    40–50 minutes.

3. Combine the mashed and cooled potatoes with the rest of the
    Smoked Salmon Fishcake ingredients.

4. Set up the flour, egg and breadcrumb bowls for both the **Smoked
    Salmon Fishcakes** and **Wiener Schnitzels** together. You should
    have 200 g flour in one bowl, 4 eggs and 1 cup of milk in another
    bowl, and 500 g breadcrumbs in the third. Dip the fish cakes
    first, before the pork, because the pork is raw. There should be
    no transfer in flavours from the fish cake to the schnitzels.

5. Form the fishcakes, coat with crumbs, and set aside in the fridge
    for frying.

6. Bash the pork for the **Wiener Schnitzels** and crumb coat.

7. Cook off the meat and herbs for the **Beef Tacos**, set aside to cool.

8. Prepare the **Sausage & Mushroom Bolognese**.

9. Prepare the **Easy Lentil Soup** and simmer for 30 minutes.

10. Increase the oven temperature to 200°C. By now the meatloaf
    should be out and cooling.

11. Throw together the **One-Pan Chicken** and bake for 45 minutes.
    (We recommend you eat this meal on the day you cook it).

12. Allow all dishes to cool completely before chilling or freezing.

Easiest Ever Meatloaf

Ingredients

oil, for greasing
1 onion, finely chopped
1 carrot, grated
300 g beef mince
300 g pork mince
90 g breadcrumbs

1 egg
2 teaspoons sweet paprika
2 teaspoons ground cumin
100 ml tomato sauce (ketchup)
1½ teaspoons salt
½ teaspoon pepper

Method

1. Preheat the oven to 180°C.
2. Grease a loaf tin with a little oil. Alternatively, use a small square lamington tin (although your meatloaf will be distinctly less loaf-shaped!).
3. Combine all of the ingredients in a large mixing bowl. Gently press the mixture into the prepared tin.
4. Bake for 40–50 minutes until cooked through and slightly caramelised on the top.

Serving Suggestion

Serve with mashed potatoes and a green salad.

Storage & Reheating

Allow to cool completely before chilling or freezing. The meatloaf will keep for up to 1 week in the fridge or up to 2 months in the freezer.

If cooking from frozen, defrost overnight in the fridge. Cover with foil and heat in a 180°C oven for about 20 minutes.

Smoked Salmon Fishcakes

Ingredients

5 large potatoes, peeled

50 g butter

2 tablespoons Dijon mustard (or your favourite variety)

1 bunch dill, leaves picked and finely chopped

1 bunch chives, finely chopped

zest of 1 lemon

400 g smoked salmon, roughly chopped

1 teaspoon salt

½ teaspoon pepper

2 eggs

½ cup milk

100 g flour

250 g breadcrumbs

oil, for shallow-frying

Method

1. Boil the potatoes in salted boiling water until cooked through. Transfer to a large bowl and add the butter and mustard. Mash thoroughly and set aside to cool.

2. Combine the herbs, lemon zest, smoked salmon, salt and pepper in a small bowl. Add to the cooled mashed potato and mix thoroughly. Divide the mixture into 8 large balls or 16 small. Flatten each ball to about 3 cm thickness.

3. Whisk the eggs and milk together in a small bowl. Place the flour in another bowl and put the breadcrumbs in a third bowl or on a plate. Coat each fishcake in flour, then dip in the egg and milk mixture, followed by the breadcrumbs, pressing gently to adhere the crumbs.

4. Set aside in the fridge for 30 minutes to firm up. Or, you can freeze from this point by placing uncooked fish cakes between layers of baking paper in an airtight container.

5. Heat a little oil in a large heavy-based saucepan over medium–high heat. Fry the fishcakes in batches for about 5–7 minutes on each side or until golden and crispy.

Serving Suggestion

Serve with a fresh green salad or lightly steamed greens.

Storage & Reheating

Allow to cool completely before chilling or freezing. If freezing uncooked, see step 4. The fishcakes will keep for 3–4 days in the fridge or 1 month in the freezer.

If cooking from frozen, defrost overnight in the fridge and follow steps 5–6 to cook.

Wiener Schnitzel

Sounds impressive and complicated but between me and you all we're doing is crumbing a bit of flattened pork and serving it with boiled potatoes. Ssshh, don't tell anyone!

Ingredients

800 g deboned pork loin, cut into
    6 pieces
2 eggs
½ cup milk
100 g flour
250 g breadcrumbs

50–80 ml oil for shallow-frying
    (depending on the size of your
    pan)
50 g butter
1 lemon, cut into wedges

Method

1. Lay out a long sheet of plastic wrap and lay the pork on top, at least 4 cm apart. Lay another sheet of plastic wrap over the top. Gently beat the pork with a rolling pin until the pieces are very thin, but without holes. Season each side with a pinch of salt and pepper.
2. Whisk the eggs and milk together in a small bowl. Place the flour in another bowl and put the breadcrumbs on a large plate. Coat each piece of pork in the flour, then dip in the egg and milk mixture, followed by the breadcrumbs. Don't press the breadcrumbs on too hard or the crumb texture will be hard rather than light and crisp.

★ **You can refrigerate or freeze the schnitzels at this stage. Place on a baking sheet lined with baking paper and freeze, before transferring to an airtight container or zip lock bag.**

3. Pour enough oil into a heavy-based frying pan to come ½ cm up the side of the pan over medium–high heat. Add the butter and cook the pork in two batches, about 1 minute on each side. Drain on kitchen paper.
4. Serve with lemon wedges on the side.

Serving Suggestion

Serve with boiled new potatoes and a green salad.

Storage & Reheating

Refrigerate or freeze uncooked schnitzels after step 2. They will keep for 5 days in the fridge or 3 months in the freezer. If cooking from frozen, defrost overnight in the fridge and follow steps 3–4 to cook.

Cooked schnitzels will keep for 1 week in the fridge or 2 months in the freezer. Allow to chill completely before transferring to the fridge or freezer.

Beef Tacos

Ingredients

1 tablespoon of oil
500 g beef mince
2 teaspoons ground cumin
2 teaspoons garlic powder
½ teaspoon chilli powder
1 tablespoon tomato paste
2 teaspoons brown sugar
1 bunch oregano, roughly chopped
salt and pepper

12 taco shells or soft flour tortillas
4 tomatoes, diced
1 avocado, flesh diced
1 bunch coriander, leaves roughly chopped
juice of 1 lime
200 g mozzarella, shredded
½ iceberg lettuce, shredded
Tabasco sauce (optional)

Method

1. Heat the olive oil in a large frying pan over medium–high heat. Add the mince and cook, stirring often, until browned and starting to crisp. Add the spices and stir through, then cook for a further couple of minutes. Add the tomato paste, brown sugar and oregano and stir through. Continue cooking for a few more minutes until the mince is cooked through. Add salt and pepper – adjust to taste.
2. Heat the taco shells or tortillas in the oven until the shells are crisp or the tortillas are soft and pliable.
3. Combine the tomato, avocado and coriander and dress with lime juice. Season to taste.
4. Let everyone dig in and help themselves. We like to build our tacos in this order: base, taco mince, grated mozzarella, a little of the 'salsa' mixture and some shredded lettuce on top. Drizzle a few drops of Tabasco sauce over the top if you like your tacos with an added spicy kick!

Storage & Reheating

Allow the taco mince to cool completely before chilling or freezing. It will keep for 1 week in the fridge or 2 months in the freezer.

If cooking from frozen, defrost overnight in the fridge. Heat the mince in the oven or in a frying pan until thoroughly heated through, adding a little water if the mixture is too dry.

Sausage & Mushroom 'Bolognese'

Ingredients

600 g good quality pork sausages, casings removed

12 button mushrooms, thinly sliced

1 tablespoon oil

1 x 700 ml jar tomato passata

100 ml red wine

3 handfuls baby spinach

Method

1. Place a large heavy-based saucepan over medium heat. As the saucepan heats up, add the sausage meat, breaking up the meat with a wooden spoon until it is brown all over.
2. Add the mushrooms and cook, stirring occasionally, for 5 minutes or until softened.
3. Add the oil and increase the heat for about 1 minute to get the mixture sizzling hot, then reduce the heat and add the passata and wine. Allow to simmer for a few minutes and then remove from the heat. Toss the spinach leaves in and stir through to wilt. Season, to taste.

Serving Suggestion

Serve sauce over al dente spaghetti and a sprinkle of grated parmesan.

Storage & Reheating

Allow to cool completely before chilling or freezing. The bolognese will keep for 1 week in the fridge or 3 months in the freezer.

If cooking from frozen, defrost overnight in the fridge. Reheat thoroughly in a medium-sized saucepan over low heat.

Easy Lentil Soup

Ingredients

3 tablespoons olive oil
1 onion, finely chopped
4 garlic cloves, finely chopped
2 carrots, finely diced
4 thyme sprigs, leaves picked
2 teaspoons ground cumin
1 cup green lentils
1 x 400 g tin whole peeled
    tomatoes

1 litre vegetable stock
2 cups water
1 teaspoon salt
½ teaspoon black pepper
4 handfuls baby spinach leaves
juice of 1 lemon

Method

1. Heat the oil in a large heavy-based saucepan over medium heat. Add the onion, garlic, carrot and thyme and cook, stirring occasionally, for about 5 minutes. Add the cumin, stir, and cook for a further 2 minutes.
2. Stir in the lentils, tinned tomatoes, stock and water. Add the salt and black pepper. Bring to the boil.
3. Reduce the heat to low and simmer for 30 minutes or until the lentils are just tender but not mushy. Set yourself a timer to help.
4. Toss the spinach leaves in at the end and stir until wilted. Season the soup to taste and add a few squeezes of lemon juice.

Serving Suggestion

Serve with hunks of crusty bread.

Storage & Reheating

Allow to cool completely before chilling or freezing. The soup will keep for 1 week in the fridge or 3 months in the freezer.

If cooking from frozen, defrost overnight in the fridge. Bring the soup to a simmer in a large saucepan, then serve.

One-Pan Chicken

We recommend you eat this meal on the day you cook it.

Ingredients

3 tablespoons olive oil

500 g chicken drumsticks

240 g chicken thighs, boneless

4 large potatoes, cut into 8 chunks

1 red onion, cut into 8 chunks

2 red capsicums, deseeded and cut
   into 10 pieces

8 garlic cloves, peeled and bashed

6 rosemary sprigs, leaves picked

6 thyme sprigs, leaves picked

1 teaspoon ground cumin

1 teaspoon ground coriander

1 teaspoon salt

1 teaspoon pepper

1 bunch parsley, leaves chopped

Method

1. Preheat the oven to 200°C.
2. Pour the olive oil into a large baking dish, tilting it to coat the base and sides. Add all of the ingredients to the dish and mix well with your hands.
3. Bake for 45 minutes or until the chicken is cooked through and the potatoes are crisp and tender.
4. Scatter over the parsley and serve.

Serving Suggestion

Serve with lightly steamed green vegetables or leafy greens.

Storage & Reheating

Allow to cool completely before chilling or freezing. This dish will keep for 1 week in the fridge or 1 month in the freezer.

If cooking from frozen, defrost overnight in the fridge. Drizzle over 1 tablespoon of olive oil and tightly cover the dish with foil. Heat the oven to 160°C and heat through for 20–25 minutes.

Oven-Baked Dinners

Oven-Baked Dinners

These are great for those weeks when all you need is some lovely comfort food every night of the week! Or, if you don't want them every night, pop them in the freezer for when that time comes.

"I set aside a Sunday morning, put on a kids' movie and made a rather large coffee.

I prepared all the meat and put them into bowls, ready to go. For me, prepping everything first was the easiest option and I felt that it made the cooking aspect run smoothly.

"Assembling the Lasagne and Shepherd's Pie was easy and they went into the oven. I decided to freeze the pie mix and pastry separately as I wanted to make individual pies using my pie maker on the day. The results were great! I defrosted the pastry and filling that morning and my five-year-old helped roll the pastry while I made the pies. Although it took a little while it was certainly easier than preparing a whole meal from scratch!

"The enchiladas were easy from start to finish as was the marinade for the pork.

Lastly, I cooked the tagine and the cannelloni. Both smelt amazing and were lucky to even make it to the freezer. I used a large zip lock bag to pipe the cannelloni which worked a treat – and no cleaning up!"

– MamaBaker, Lauren

Menu

Lasagne

Shepherd's Pie

Baked Chicken Tagine

Chicken Enchiladas

Four Cheese & Broccoli Cannelloni

Eggplant Parmigiana

Asian Salmon

Shopping List

Meat & Fish	Fruit & Veg	Dairy & Frozen
1 kg beef mince 1 kg chicken breasts 1 kg skinless chicken thighs, boneless 800 g salmon fillet	3 onions 2 heads garlic 6 cm piece ginger 4–5 large potatoes 7 carrots 1 bunch celery 2 heads broccoli 3 large eggplants 2 long green chillies 1 bunch mint 1 bunch thyme 1 bunch oregano 1 bunch basil 1 lemon	2¼ cups milk 100 g butter 5 eggs 650 g mozzarella 200 g parmesan 100 g tasty cheese 400 g ricotta 75 g feta 2 cups frozen peas
Tins, Jars & Dry Goods	**Pantry Essentials**	**Other Ingredients**
5 x 400 g tin whole peeled tomatoes 1 x 400 g tin crushed tomatoes 1 x 400 g tin black beans 2 cups breadcrumbs	olive oil canola, sunflower or grapeseed oil 1.5 litres chicken stock 50 g flour 9 tbs tomato paste ½ cup honey 1¼ tbs brown sugar salt pepper 1 tbs mustard 3 tbs soy sauce 2 tbs sesame oil 2 tsp paprika 1 tsp chilli powder 1 whole nutmeg or 1 tsp ground nutmeg 3 tsp ground cumin 2 tsp ground cinnamon	¾ cup orange juice 2 x 375 g pack fresh lasagne sheets 10–12 soft flour tortillas

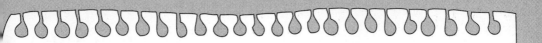

Serving Size
Each meal serves a family of 4 (approximately)

Preparation time
3½ hours

Equipment
Preparation: sharp knives, chopping boards suitable for vegetables and fruit, meat and fish, kitchen scales, measuring cups and spoons, vegetable peeler, grater, citrus zester, mixing bowls in assorted sizes, potato masher, whisk, mixing spoons, plastic wrap, paper towel.

Cooking: large, heavy-based frying pan, medium-sized frying pan, medium and large saucepans, casserole dish, baking dishes (disposable aluminium baking dishes are handy when bulk cooking).

Storage: zip lock bags, airtight containers suitable for freezing, foil.

Storage & Reheating
All of these meals are freezer-friendly and will need to be defrosted before you plan to eat them. Don't panic if you forget to do it the night before and remember in the morning, just defrost them on the kitchen bench until dinnertime.

If you can't wait and are going to tee them up for the next couple of nights, then they can be popped in the fridge for a couple of days until you're ready to cook them.

Once-A-Week Cooking Preparation

	Total	Lasagne	Shepherd's Pie	Baked Chicken Tagine
Fresh Produce				
Onions	3	1 finely chopped	1 finely chopped	
Garlic heads	2	3 cloves, finely chopped	3 cloves, finely chopped	6 cloves, finely chopped
Ginger	6 cm piece			4 cm piece, grated
Potatoes	4–5		4–5, peeled and cut into 4	
Carrots	7	3 finely diced	4 finely diced	
Celery	1	3 stalks, finely diced	4 stalks, finely diced	
Broccoli	2			
Eggplant	3			
Green chillies	2			
Mint	1			½ bunch, finely chopped
Thyme	1			6 sprigs, leaves picked
Oregano	1			
Basil	1			
Lemon	1			1 quartered
Cheese				
Mozzarella	650 g			
Tasty	100 g			
Parmesan	200 g	100 g, grated		
Feta	75 g			
Meat				
Beef mince	1 kg	reserve 500 g	reserve 500 g	
Chicken breasts	1 kg			
Chicken thighs, boneless	1 kg			cut in half
Salmon	800 g			

Chicken Enchiladas	Four Cheese & Broccoli Cannelloni	Eggplant Parmigiana	Asian Salmon
1 finely sliced			
	4 cloves, finely chopped	4 cloves, finely chopped	2 cloves, finely chopped
			2 cm piece, finely chopped
	2 heads, florets chopped, stalks peeled and finely chopped		
		3 sliced 1 cm thick	
2 deseeded and finely sliced			
2 sprigs, leaves picked		8 sprigs, leaves picked	
		1 bunch, half roughly chopped	
250 g, grated	100 g, grated	300 g, grated	
	100 g, grated		
		100 g, grated	
	75 g, crumbled		
diced into 3-cm pieces			
			pin bone fillet, if necessary, and slice into 4 pieces

Once-A-Week Cooking Plan

Ovens vary greatly in their capacity so you may be unable to bake all these dishes in the one cooking session. If this is the case, we recommend that you either store the prepared meal uncooked in the fridge for a couple of days (please see recipe instructions) until you're ready to cook it, or simply freeze uncooked.

1. Preheat the oven to 180°C.

2. Prepare the meat bases for the **Lasagne** and the **Shepherd's Pie** first as they require longer cooking time.

3. Make the topping for the **Shepherd's Pie**.

4. Prepare the chicken for the **Baked Chicken Tagine** and place in the oven if cooking that day.

5. Make the filling for the **Chicken Enchiladas**. Fill the tortillas and top with the sauce. Place in the oven if cooking that day.

6. Make the filling and the sauce for the **Four Cheese & Broccoli Cannelloni**. Fill and roll the pasta sheets and top with the sauce. Place in the oven if cooking that day.

7. Prepare the sauce for the **Eggplant Parmigiana**. Coat and fry the eggplant and form the layers. Place in the oven if cooking that day.

8. Put together the **Shepherd's Pie** and place in the oven if cooking that day.

9. Make the béchamel for the **Lasagne**, put the layers together and place in the oven if cooking that day.

10. Marinate and refrigerate or freeze the **Asian Salmon**.

11. Allow all dishes to cool completely before chilling or freezing.

Lasagne

Ingredients

2 tablespoons oil
1 onion, finely chopped
3 carrots, finely diced
3 celery stalks, finely diced
3 garlic cloves, finely chopped
500 g beef mince

100 ml tomato paste
1 x 400 g tin whole peeled
  tomatoes
2 cups chicken stock
375 g pack fresh lasagne sheets

Béchamel sauce

50 g butter
50 g flour
2 cups milk

½ teaspoon freshly grated nutmeg
  or ½ teaspoon ground nutmeg
salt and pepper
100 g parmesan, grated

Method

1. Heat the oil in a large heavy-based saucepan over medium heat. Sauté the onion, carrot and celery, stirring often, until the onion is translucent. Add the garlic and cook for a further 10 minutes.
2. Add the mince and cook for 5–7 minutes, using a wooden spoon to break up any clumps. Stir through the tomato paste and cook for a further 2–3 minutes. Add the tomatoes and chicken stock.
3. Leave to simmer, covered, for 30 minutes, and then remove the lid for final 30 minutes.
4. When you are ready to assemble the lasagne, make the béchamel. Melt the butter in a small saucepan. When it is frothing, add the flour and cook for a couple of minutes until the mixture resembles wet sand.
5. Gradually add the milk, whisking continuously to prevent lumps forming. Bring to the boil and boil for at least 2–3 minutes, but keep whisking! Once thickened to a mayonnaise-like consistency, remove from the heat and season with the nutmeg and salt and pepper, to taste.
6. Preheat the oven to 180°C.

7. Layer the sauce and the lasagne sheets in a greased baking dish, starting with the sauce and finishing with a layer of pasta. Top with the béchamel sauce and parmesan.
8. Bake for 30–40 minutes or until the top is golden and bubbling.

Serving Suggestion
Serve with a fresh green salad and garlic bread.

Storage & Reheating
Allow to cool completely before chilling or freezing. The lasagne will keep for 1 week in the fridge or 2 months in the freezer.

If cooking from frozen, defrost overnight in the fridge. Cover with foil and bake for 20–30 minutes at 180°C or until heated through and the cheese is bubbling again.

Shepherd's Pie

Traditionally, Shepherd's Pie uses lamb mince but we've used beef mince here because it's easier to get hold of and probably cheaper too. If you would prefer lamb, simply substitute the beef in this recipe.

Ingredients

2 tablespoons oil

1 onion, finely chopped

4 carrots, finely diced

4 celery stalks, finely diced

3 garlic cloves, finely chopped

500 g beef mince

2 tablespoons tomato paste

700 ml chicken stock

2 cups frozen peas

Mashed potato topping

4–5 large potatoes, peeled and quartered

¼ cup milk

3 tablespoons butter

Method

1. Heat the oil in a large saucepan over medium heat. Add the onion, carrot and celery and cook, stirring often, for 10 minutes. Add the garlic and cook for a further 5 minutes.
2. Add the mince and cook for 8–10 minutes, breaking up any clumps with a wooden spoon. Add the tomato paste and cook for a further 2–3 minutes. Stir in the stock. Simmer, uncovered, for 45 minutes.
3. Season with salt and pepper to taste. Add the frozen peas to the mixture and stir through. The residual heat will cook them through.
4. Preheat the oven to 180°C
5. To make the mashed potato topping, boil the potatoes in salted boiling water until tender. Remove from the heat and add the milk and butter. Mash the potatoes and season with salt and pepper.
6. Spoon the beef mixture into a deep casserole dish and top with the mashed potato.
7. Cook for 20–30 minutes or until mashed potato is golden and centre is hot.

Serving Suggestion

Serve with steamed vegetables.

Storage & Reheating

Allow to cool completely before chilling or freezing. This dish will keep for 1 week in the fridge or 2 months in the freezer.

If cooking from frozen, defrost overnight in the fridge. Place the pie in a cold oven and heat to 180°C. Once the temperature reaches 180°C, cook the pie for 20 minutes or until crisp on top and heated through.

Baked Chicken Tagine

Ingredients

1 kg skinless chicken thighs, boneless, halved

1 tablespoon olive oil

1 tablespoon butter

6 garlic cloves, finely chopped

6 thyme sprigs, leaves picked

¼ bunch mint, leaves chopped

1½ cups chicken stock

Dry rub

4 cm piece ginger, grated

2 teaspoons ground cumin

2 teaspoons ground cinnamon

2 teaspoons paprika

1 teaspoon salt

¼ bunch mint, leaves chopped

Glaze

½ cup honey

¾ cup orange juice

1 lemon, quartered

Method

1. Preheat the oven to 180°C. Lightly grease a ceramic or glass baking dish.
2. To make the rub, combine the ginger, cumin, cinnamon, paprika, salt and mint in a large bowl. Add the chicken thighs and toss to coat well with the rub (if you have time, cover and place in the fridge for up to an hour for the flavours to infuse).
3. Heat the oil and butter in a large frying pan over medium–high heat. Brown the chicken on all sides or until starting to caramelise and colour – this will take about 4 minutes. Transfer the chicken to the baking dish.
4. Add the garlic to the pan and cook for one minute. Scatter this over the chicken, along with the thyme and the mint, then pour in the chicken stock.
5. Bake for 35–45 minutes or until the chicken is cooked through.
6. To make the glaze, place the honey, orange juice and lemon quarters in a small saucepan over low heat. Simmer for around 10 minutes, or until the glaze is reduced and thickened.

7. Remove the chicken from the oven and pour off any excess liquid (you can keep this to use as stock in a soup).
8. Pour the glaze over the meat. Cover with foil and bake for a further 20–25 minutes.

Serving Suggestion
Serve with couscous and slivered almonds.

Storage & Reheating
Allow to cool completely before chilling or freezing. The baked chicken will keep for 1 week in the fridge or 2 months in the freezer.

If cooking from frozen, defrost overnight in the fridge or on the morning of the day you wish to cook it. Cover with foil and bake for 20–25 minutes at 180°C or until heated through.

Chicken Enchiladas

Enchiladas are a delicious Mexican meal of tortillas stuffed with meat (or whatever you like!), covered with a chilli sauce and baked.

Ingredients

1 x 400 g tin crushed tomatoes
2 tablespoons tomato paste
1 teaspoon chilli powder
1 teaspoon ground cumin
small handful oregano leaves
½ teaspoon salt
2 tablespoons oil
1 onion, finely sliced

2 long green chillies, deseeded and finely sliced
1 kg chicken breasts, diced into 3 cm pieces
1 x 400 g tin black beans
10–12 soft flour tortillas
250 g mozzarella, grated

Method

1. Grease a ceramic or glass baking dish.
2. Place the tomatoes, tomato paste, chilli powder, ground cumin, oregano and salt in a small saucepan and bring to the boil. Set aside.
3. Heat the oil in a large frying pan over medium–high heat. Add the onion and sauté until translucent. Add the chillies along with the chicken breast and cook for about 8 minutes, or until chicken is browned and cooked through. Remove from the heat.
4. Drain and rinse the black beans. Lay out the tortillas on a clean work surface.
5. Preheat the oven to 200°C.
6. Spoon 1 tablespoon of sauce on a tortilla. Add 2 tablespoons of beans down the middle, add some chicken, then sprinkle with a little cheese. Roll it up and place in the greased dish. Repeat with the remaining ingredients, setting aside a little of the cheese to sprinkle over the top.
7. Pour the sauce over the rolled tortillas and sprinkle with the remaining cheese.
8. Bake for 20–30 minutes until the sauce is bubbling and the cheese is golden.

Serving Suggestion
Serve with a green salad.

Storage & Reheating
Allow to cool completely before chilling or freezing. The enchiladas will keep for 1 week in the fridge or 2 months in the freezer.

If cooking from frozen, defrost overnight in the fridge or on the kitchen bench the morning of the day you wish to cook it. Cover with foil and bake for 20 minutes at 180°C or until heated through and the cheese is bubbling again.

Four Cheese & Broccoli Cannelloni

Ingredients

2 x 400 g tins whole peeled
  tomatoes

1 teaspoon sugar

4 garlic cloves, finely chopped

2 tablespoons olive oil

2 heads broccoli, florets chopped,
  stalk peeled and finely
  chopped

400 g ricotta

75 g feta, crumbled

100 g tasty cheese, grated

100 g mozzarella, grated

2 eggs, lightly beaten

½ teaspoon ground nutmeg

375 g fresh lasagne sheets

Method

1. Preheat oven to 200°C. Grease a large glass baking dish.
2. Place the tinned tomatoes, sugar and half of the garlic in a saucepan over medium heat. Simmer, stirring occasionally, until reduced by one-third, about 10 minutes. Pour half of the tomato mixture in the baking dish and spread evenly.
3. Heat the olive oil in a large saucepan and place over medium heat. Sauté the broccoli with the remaining garlic until tender. Transfer to a large bowl and set aside to cool.
4. Combine the broccoli and garlic with the ricotta, feta, and half of the tasty cheese and mozzarella. Add the egg, nutmeg and mix well. Season with salt and pepper, to taste.
5. Lay out the pasta sheets, place 2 tablespoons of the broccoli and cheese mixture at the base of each sheet and roll up into tubes. Place the cannelloni in the baking dish on top of the sauce. Top with the remaining sauce and cheese.
6. Bake for 30 minutes. Cover with foil and bake for a further 15 minutes.

Serving Suggestion

Serve with fresh green salad.

Storage & Reheating

Allow to cool completely before chilling or freezing. The cannelloni will keep for 1 week in the fridge or 2 months in the freezer.

If cooking from frozen, defrost overnight in the fridge or on the kitchen bench the day you wish to cook it. Cover with foil and bake for 15–20 minutes at 180°C or until heated through.

Eggplant Parmigiana

Ingredients

2 x 400 g tins whole peeled
  tomatoes
4 garlic cloves, finely chopped
1 teaspoon brown sugar
1 bunch basil, leaves picked, half
  roughly chopped
8 oregano sprigs, leaves picked

3 eggs, beaten
2 cups breadcrumbs
3 large eggplants, sliced 1 cm
  thick
300 g mozzarella, grated
100 g parmesan, grated
4 tablespoons olive oil

Method

1. Preheat the oven to 180°C. Lightly grease a glass or ceramic baking dish and two baking trays.
2. In a small saucepan, add the tinned tomatoes, garlic, brown sugar, the chopped basil leaves and a pinch of the oregano leaves. Bring to the boil and allow to simmer, stirring, for about 10 minutes. Remove from the heat and set aside.
3. Place the beaten eggs and breadcrumbs in separate bowls. Dip each slice of eggplant into the egg and then the breadcrumbs. Transfer to one of the greased baking trays and repeat with the remaining eggplant.
4. Bake for 10 minutes. Flip each piece and then bake for a further 5 minutes or until golden brown.
5. Spread half the sauce in the baking dish, then add a layer of the baked eggplant and half of the remaining basil and oregano. Top with half of the grated cheese, then repeat with the remaining ingredients.
6. Bake for 30 minutes until heated through and the cheese is golden.

Serving Suggestion

Serve with a fresh salad or steamed vegetables.

Storage & Reheating

Allow to cool completely before chilling or freezing. This dish will keep for up to 1 week in the fridge or 2 months in the freezer.

If cooking from frozen, defrost overnight in the fridge or on the kitchen bench the day you wish to cook it. Cover with foil and bake for 20 minutes at 180°C or until heated through and the cheese is bubbling.

Asian Salmon

Ingredients

2 garlic cloves, finely chopped

2 cm piece ginger, finely chopped

1 tablespoon wholegrain mustard

3 tablespoons soy sauce

2 tablespoons sesame oil

1 tablespoon brown sugar

800 g salmon fillet, sliced into 4 pieces

Method

1. To make the marinade, whisk the garlic, ginger, mustard, soy sauce, sesame oil and sugar in a large bowl. Place the salmon fillets in the marinade and set aside for 10 minutes.

* **You can refrigerate or freeze the salmon at this stage. Put all of the ingredients into a large zip lock bag and place in the fridge or freezer.**

2. Preheat the oven to 180°C.
3. Place the fish and marinade in an oven-proof ceramic or glass baking dish.
4. Bake for 15–20 minutes or until the fish feels firm when pressed at its thickest point.

Serving Suggestion

Serve with steamed rice scattered with sliced spring onions.

Storage & Reheating

If freezing at step 1, can be frozen for up to 2 months.

If freezing after step 4, allow to cool completely before storing.

Once cooked, if storing in the fridge, eat within two days.

If you plan to eat the fish within 2 days of purchase, store the marinated fish in the fridge. Otherwise, store in the freezer for up to 2 months.

If cooking from frozen, defrost overnight in the fridge. Follow steps 2–4 to cook.

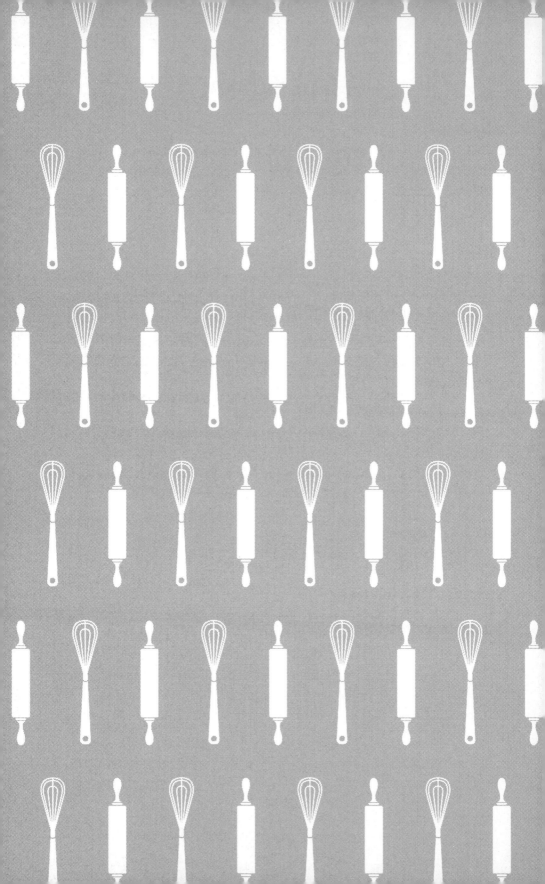

Nourishing Slow Cooker Comfort Meals

Nourishing Slow Cooker Comfort Meals

As the temperature begins to drop, there's nothing quite like coming home after a long day to the comforting aromas of a nourishing family dinner that's been doing its thing in the slow cooker all day. Change into something more comfortable, pop on your favourite family movie and enjoy a warming meal, every night of the week!

The Slow Cooker Baggie Method

With our slow cooker plans you will notice there is not the usual Once-A-Week Cooking Plan section because we use our famed Baggie Method. This is where you pop all the meal ingredients into a large zip lock baggie, freeze it and then pull it out of the freezer when you're ready to cook it up.

You will find specific Baggie instructions underneath each individual recipe.

Here's how it works:

- Get 7 large zip lock baggies. Label each baggie with the name of the dish it will contain and the date of preparation. Also, add the cooking time and temperature that the slow cooker should be set to.
- Place each labelled baggie into one of 7 large bowls.
- Fill each labelled baggie with the ingredients as you prepare them. (For example, divide the chopped onions among baggies for dishes that contain chopped onion.)
- Refer to the recipes to see what other ingredients need to be added to each baggie before sealing and freezing.

Menu

Roast Beef with Carrots

Ham & White Beans

Chinese Beef & Broccoli

Lemon Pepper Chicken with Rice

Honey Mustard Chicken

Tomato, Vegetable & Barley Soup

Old-School Marinara Sauce

Shopping List

Meat & Fish	Fruit & Veg	Dairy & Frozen
1 kg beef chuck steak 1 kg ham hocks 750 g flank steak 1.2 kg chicken thighs, boneless, 1.2 kg chicken breasts	13 cloves garlic 4 onions 11 carrots 2 heads broccoli 4 large handfuls green beans 1 lemon 1 bunch rosemary 1 bunch thyme 1 bunch parsley 1 bunch basil	1 cup frozen peas

Tins, Jars & Dry Goods	Pantry Essentials	Other Ingredients
3 x 400 g tins whole peeled tomatoes 4 x 400 g cans crushed tomatoes 550 g dried white beans 1½ cups brown rice ½ cup pearl barley	olive oil 1 litre beef stock 1 litre vegetable stock 2 tbs cornstarch 2 tbs red wine vinegar ⅓ cup brown sugar ½ cup honey salt pepper ½ cup light soy sauce ½ cup mustard 1 tablespoon sesame oil 1 tsp smoked paprika 1 tbs dried dill	

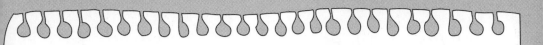

Serving Size
Each meal serves a family of 4–6

Preparation time
1.5 hours

Equipment
Slow cooker (minimum 5-litre), sharp knives, chopping boards suitable for vegetables and fruit, meat and fish, kitchen scales, measuring cups and spoons, vegetable peeler, large mixing bowls and large zip lock bags.

Storage & Reheating
While you can generally keep meat and vegetables in the fridge for the week, because these meals have combined ingredients it is necessary to freeze them straightaway. You can keep the meal you plan to cook the next day and the day after that in the fridge, but the rest should be frozen as soon as you have prepared them.

Defrost each meal overnight and pop in the slow cooker the following day. Once the meals are cooked, leftovers will keep, refrigerated, for 5–7 days. Cooked meals can also be frozen. When you defrost a cooked meal, ensure that you reheat the meal thoroughly.

Once-A-Week Cooking Preparation

	Total	Roast Beef with Carrots	Ham & White Beans	Chinese Beef & Broccoli
Dry Goods				
Cannellini beans or white beans	550 g		Soak 450 g overnight or in just-boiled water for at least 1–2 hours.	
Fresh Produce				
Garlic	1	4 cloves, thinly sliced	3 cloves, finely chopped	3 cloves, finely chopped
Onions	4		1 chopped	
Carrots	11	6 sliced		
Broccoli	2			2 heads, florets chopped, stalk peeled and cut into batons
Green beans (handfuls)	4			
Lemon	1			
Rosemary	1	4 sprigs, leaves finely chopped		
Thyme	1			
Parsley	1			
Basil	1			
Meat				
Flank steak	750 g			sliced into 5 cm-long pieces
Chicken thighs, boneless	1.2 kg			
Chicken breasts	1.2 kg			

Lemon Pepper Chicken with Rice	Honey Mustard Chicken	Tomato, Vegetable & Barley Soup	Old-School Marinara Sauce
		soak 100 g overnight	
			3 cloves, finely chopped
1 finely chopped		1 chopped	1 finely chopped
1 sliced		4 diced	
2 large handfuls, topped and tailed		2 large handfuls, topped and tailed and cut in half	
1 thinly sliced			
3 sprigs, leaves finely chopped		3 sprigs, leaves finely chopped	
		1 bunch, leaves finely chopped	
			½ bunch, leaves finely chopped
cut into 3 pieces each			
	butterflied		

Roast Beef with Carrots

Ingredients

6 carrots, sliced

4 garlic cloves, thinly sliced

4 rosemary sprigs, leaves finely chopped

1 kg beef chuck steak

3 tablespoons olive oil

2 tablespoons red wine vinegar

3 cups beef stock

1 teaspoon salt

½ teaspoon black pepper

Method

Place a large zip lock bag in a large bowl and add all the ingredients to the bag. Squeeze out as much air as possible and seal. Give the bag a good shake. It is now ready to freeze.

To Cook

1. Defrost the zip lock bag overnight in the fridge then empty the ingredients into a slow cooker.
2. Cook for 8–10 hours on LOW.

Serving Suggestion

Boil and mash some potatoes to your liking and serve on the side.

Storage & Reheating

Once this dish is cooked, leftovers will keep for 5–7 days in the fridge and 2–3 months in the freezer. Cooked meals can be frozen. Cool completely before chilling or freezing.

If cooking from frozen, defrost overnight in the fridge, then reheat the meal thoroughly in a microwave or covered saucepan.

Ham & White Beans

Ingredients

450 g dried white beans, soaked
    in water overnight
1 onion, chopped
3 garlic cloves, finely chopped

1 kg ham hocks
1 teaspoon salt
½ teaspoon pepper

Method

Drain the white beans and place in a zip lock bag along with the other ingredients. Squeeze out as much air as possible and seal. Give the bag a good shake. It is now ready to freeze.

To cook

1. Defrost the zip lock bag overnight in the fridge then empty the ingredients into a slow cooker along with 1.5 litres water.
2. Cook for 8–10 hours on LOW until the beans are tender and the ham is soft.
3. Remove the hocks and shred the meat from the bones before returning to the pot and mixing through.

Serving Suggestion

Serve with crusty bread on the side.

Storage & Reheating

Once this dish is cooked, leftovers will keep for 5–7 days in the fridge and 2–3 months in the freezer. Cooked meals can be frozen. Cool completely before chilling or freezing.

If cooking from frozen, defrost overnight in the fridge, then reheat the meal thoroughly in a microwave or covered saucepan.

Chinese Beef & Broccoli

Ingredients

750 g flank steak, sliced into
5 cm-long pieces

3 garlic cloves, peeled and finely
chopped

½ cup light soy sauce

⅓ cup brown sugar

1 tablespoon sesame oil

1 cup beef stock

2 tablespoons cornstarch

2 broccoli heads, florets chopped,
stalk peeled and cut into batons

Method

Place a zip lock bag in a large bowl and add all of the ingredients except
the stock, cornstarch and broccoli. Squeeze out as much air as possible
and seal. Give the bag a good shake. It is now ready to freeze.

To Cook

1. Defrost the zip lock bag overnight in the fridge then empty the
   ingredients into a slow cooker along with the beef stock.
2. Cook for 5–6 hours on LOW.
3. Once cooked, whisk together the cornstarch and 4 tablespoons
   water to make a slurry. Add this to the slow cooker and stir.
4. Add the broccoli and cook for an additional 10 minutes until the
   sauce is thickened.

Serving Suggestion

Serve with basmati rice on the side.

Storage & Reheating

Once this dish is cooked, leftovers will keep for 5–7 days in the fridge
and 2–3 months in the freezer. Cooked meals can be frozen. Cool
completely before chilling or freezing.

If cooking from frozen, defrost overnight in the fridge, then reheat
the meal thoroughly in a microwave or saucepan.

Lemon Pepper Chicken with Rice

Ingredients

1 onion, finely chopped

1 carrot, sliced

2 large handfuls green beans, topped and tailed

1 lemon, thinly sliced

3 thyme sprigs, leaves finely chopped

6 chicken thighs, boneless, each cut into 3 pieces

1½ cups brown rice

1 teaspoon salt

1 teaspoon black pepper

Method

Place a zip lock bag in a large bowl and add all of the ingredients to the bag. Squeeze out as much air as possible and seal. Give the bag a good shake. It is now ready to freeze.

To Cook

1. Defrost the zip lock bag overnight in the fridge then empty the ingredients into a slow cooker.
2. Add 2 cups water and cook for 6–8 hours on LOW.
3. Discard the lemon slices and serve.

Serving Suggestion

Serve with lightly steamed buttered broccoli.

Storage & Reheating

Once this dish is cooked, leftovers will keep for 5–7 days in the fridge and 2–3 months in the freezer. Cooked meals can be frozen. Cool completely before chilling or freezing.

If cooking from frozen, defrost overnight in the fridge, then reheat the meal thoroughly in a microwave or saucepan.

Honey Mustard Chicken

Ingredients

4 large chicken breasts, butterflied
½ cup honey
½ cup Dijon mustard
1 teaspoon smoked paprika

1 tablespoon dried dill
½ teaspoon salt
black pepper

Method

Place a zip lock bag in a large bowl and add all of the ingredients to the bag. Squeeze out as much air as possible and seal. Give the bag a good shake. It is now ready to freeze.

To Cook

1. Defrost the zip lock bag overnight in the fridge then empty the ingredients into a slow cooker.
2. Cook for 6–8 hours on LOW.

Serving Suggestion

Serve with some mashed potatoes and a green salad.

Storage & Reheating

Once this dish is cooked, leftovers will keep for 5–7 days in the fridge and 2–3 months in the freezer. Cooked meals can be frozen. Cool completely before chilling or freezing.

If cooking from frozen, defrost overnight in the fridge, then reheat the meal thoroughly in a microwave or saucepan.

Tomato, Vegetable & Barley Soup

Ingredients

100 g dried white beans, soaked in water overnight

1 onion, chopped

4 carrots, diced

2 handfuls green beans, topped and tailed and cut in half

3 thyme sprigs, leaves finely chopped

1 bunch parsley, leaves finely chopped

3 x 400 g tins whole peeled tomatoes

1 cup frozen peas

½ cup pearl barley

1 teaspoon salt

½ teaspoon pepper

1 litre vegetable stock (or chicken or beef stock)

Method

Drain the beans and place in a zip lock bag along with all the ingredients except the stock. Squeeze out as much air as possible and seal. Give the bag a good shake. It is now ready to freeze.

To Cook

1. Defrost the zip lock bag overnight in the fridge then empty the ingredients into a slow cooker. Alternatively, you can cook this dish from frozen – you may need to adjust cooking time depending on your slow cooker – until soup is reheated thoroughly.
2. Add the stock, then cook for 8 hours on LOW.

Serving Suggestion

Serve with crusty bread.

Storage & Reheating

Once this dish is cooked, leftovers will keep for 5–7 days in the fridge. Cooked meals can be frozen. Cool completely before chilling or freezing.

If reheating from cooked and frozen, defrost overnight in the fridge, then reheat the meal thoroughly in a microwave or saucepan.

Old-School Marinara Sauce

This beautiful classic recipe requires barely any attention from you and will be rich and delicious from a long, slow cook.

Ingredients

1 onion, finely chopped

3 garlic cloves, finely chopped

½ bunch basil, leaves picked and finely chopped

4 x 400 g tins crushed tomatoes

¼ cup olive oil

salt and pepper to taste

Method

Place a zip lock bag in a large bowl and add all of the ingredients to the bag. Squeeze out as much air as possible and seal. Give the bag a good shake. You can keep the bag in the fridge rather than the freezer if it will be cooked within a week; otherwise, freeze.

To Cook

1. Defrost the zip lock bag overnight in the fridge then empty the ingredients into a slow cooker along with 1 cup water.
2. Cook for 5–6 hours on LOW.

Serving Suggestion

Serve with pasta topped with parmesan and chopped fresh basil leaves.

Storage & Reheating

Once this dish is cooked, leftovers will keep for 5–7 days in the fridge and 2–3 months in the freezer. If you will consume this dish within a week, there is no need to freeze. The cooked sauce can be frozen. Cool completely before chilling or freezing.

If cooking from frozen, defrost overnight in the fridge, then reheat the meal thoroughly in a microwave or saucepan.

Slow Cooker Meals with a Gourmet Twist!

Slow Cooker Meals with a Gourmet Twist!

Think all slow cooker meals are bland and boring? Think again! We've taken some restaurant favourites and given them the MamaBake Once-A-Week Slow Cook treatment! Full of flavour and texture, this menu just might change your mind about slow cooked dinners.

The Slow Cooker Baggie Method

With our slow cooker plans you will notice there is not the usual Once-A-Week Cooking Plan section because we use our famed Baggie Method. This is where you pop all the meal ingredients into a large zip lock baggie, freeze it and then pull it out of the freezer when you're ready to cook it up.

You will find specific Baggie instructions underneath each individual recipe.

Here's how it works:

- Get 7 large zip lock baggies. Label each baggie with the name of the dish it will contain and the date of preparation. Also, add the cooking time and temperature that the slow cooker should be set to.
- Place each labelled baggie into one of 7 large bowls.
- Fill each labelled baggie with the ingredients as you prepare them. (For example, divide the chopped onions among baggies for dishes that contain chopped onion.)
- Refer to the recipes to see what other ingredients need to be added to each baggie before sealing and freezing.

Menu

Braised Beef Ragù

Cashew Chicken

Easy Asian Chicken & Rice Soup

Boston Beans

Slow Cooker Pork Pot Roast

Short-Cut Jambalaya

Coconut Chicken Curry

Shopping List

Meat & Fish	Fruit & Veg	Dairy & Frozen
1.2 kg beef chuck or rump steak 1.8 kg chicken breasts 1.3 kg chicken thighs, boneless 3 smoked sausages (such as chorizo) 1.5 kg pork loin roast 5 rashers smoky bacon	6 onions 2 heads garlic 8 cm piece ginger 2 sweet potatoes 6 carrots 1 green capsicum 1 red capsicum bunch celery 1 bunch rosemary 2 bunches coriander 1 bunch parsley	none

Tins, Jars & Dry Goods	Pantry Essentials	Other Ingredients
6 x 400 g tins whole peeled tomatoes 1 cup raw cashews 1 cup basmati rice 1½ cups long-grain rice 400 ml tin coconut milk 400 g dried cannellini or white beans	olive oil canola, sunflower or grapeseed oil 2 litres chicken stock 1 jar tomato paste 2 tbs cider vinegar 3 tbs cornstarch ¼ cup plus 2 tbs plus 1 tbs brown sugar ¼ cup molasses salt black pepper ½ cup plus 2 tsp light soy sauce 4 tbs mirin 2 tbs chilli sauce 3 tbs plus 1 tsp smoked paprika ½ tsp cayenne pepper 1 tsp dried oregano 2 tsp ground cumin 1 tbs garam masala 1 tbs curry powder 2 bay leaves	¾ cup red wine

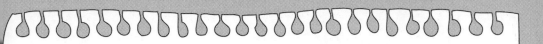

Serving Size
Each meal serves 4–6 people

Preparation time
1.5 hours

Equipment
Slow cooker (minimum 5-litre), sharp knives, chopping boards suitable for vegetables and fruit, meat and fish, kitchen scales, measuring cups and spoons, vegetable peeler, food processor or blender, large mixing bowls and large zip lock bags.

Storage & Reheating
While you can generally keep meat and vegetables in the fridge for the week, because these meals have combined ingredients it is necessary to freeze them straight away. You can keep the meal you plan to cook the next day and the day after that in the fridge, but the rest should be put in the freezer.

Defrost each meal overnight and pop in the slow cooker the following day. Once the meals are cooked, leftovers will keep, refrigerated, for 5–7 days. Cooked meals can also be frozen. When you defrost a cooked meal, ensure that you reheat the meal thoroughly.

Once-A-Week Cooking Preparation

	Total	Braised Beef Ragù	Cashew Chicken	Easy Asian Chicken & Rice Soup
Dry Good				
Cannellini beans or white beans	400 g			
Fresh Produce				
Onions	6	1 finely chopped		1 chopped
Garlic	2	3 cloves, finely chopped	2 cloves, finely chopped	4 cloves, finely chopped
Ginger	8 cm piece		4 cm piece, finely chopped	4 cm piece, finely chopped
Sweet potatoes	2			
Carrots	6			2 diced
Capsicum	2			
Celery	1			3 stalks, diced
Rosemary	1	2 sprigs, leaves finely chopped		
Coriander	2			1 bunch, stalks and roots finely chopped, leaves picked off
Parsley	1			
Meat				
Beef chuck or rump steak	1.2 kg	diced into 2-cm cubes		
Chicken thighs, boneless	1.3 kg			300 g, sliced into 3-cm pieces
Chicken breasts	1.8 kg		1 kg, diced into 3-cm cubes	300 g, sliced into 3-cm pieces
Smoked sausages	3			
Bacon	5			

Boston Beans	Slow Cooker Pork Pot Roast	Short-Cut Jambalaya	Coconut Chicken Curry
Soak overnight or in just-boiled water for at least 1–2 hours			
1 chopped	1 chopped	1 chopped	1 roughly chopped
3 cloves, finely chopped	4 cloves, finely chopped	4 cloves, finely chopped	3 cloves, roughly chopped
			2 peeled and diced into 3 cm-cubes
	4 cut into large dice		
		1 green, diced	1 red, sliced into 1 cm-long strips
		3 stalks, diced	
			1 bunch, stalks and roots blended, leaves picked off
		1 bunch, leaves finely chopped	
		500 g, diced into 2-cm cubes	500 g, diced into 3-cm cubes
			500 g, diced into 3-cm cubes
		thinly sliced	
thinly sliced			

Braised Beef Ragù

Ingredients

1.2 kg beef chuck or rump steak, diced into 2 cm cubes

3 garlic cloves, finely chopped

1 onion, finely chopped

2 rosemary sprigs, leaves finely chopped

4 x 400 g tins whole peeled tomatoes

3 tablespoons tomato paste

2 bay leaves

¾ cup red wine

2 tablespoons olive oil

2 teaspoons salt

1 teaspoon black pepper

Method

Place a zip lock bag in a large bowl and add all of the ingredients to the bag. Squeeze out as much air as possible and seal. Give the bag a good shake. It is now ready to freeze.

To Cook

1. Defrost the zip lock bag overnight in the fridge then empty the ingredients into a slow cooker.
2. Cook for 7–8 hours on LOW.

Serving Suggestion

Serve with buttered polenta.

Storage & Reheating

Once this dish is cooked, leftovers will keep for 5–7 days in the fridge and 2–3 months in the freezer. Cooked meals can be frozen. Cool completely before chilling or freezing.

If cooking from frozen, defrost overnight in the fridge, then reheat the meal thoroughly in a microwave or saucepan.

Cashew Chicken

Ingredients

1 kg chicken breasts, diced into 3-cm cubes

3 tablespoons cornstarch (or potato or tapioca starch)

2 garlic cloves finely chopped

4 cm piece ginger, finely chopped

½ cup light soy sauce

4 tablespoons mirin

4 tablespoons tomato paste

2 tablespoons chilli sauce

2 tablespoons brown sugar

1 tablespoon oil

½ teaspoon black pepper

1 cup raw cashews

Method

1. Coat the chicken with the cornstarch.
2. Combine the sauce ingredients in a large bowl and whisk.
3. If you prefer your cashews crunchy, do not add them until the end of cooking. If you like tender cashews, add them with the other ingredients.
4. Place the zip lock bag in a large bowl and add all of the ingredients to the bag. Squeeze out as much air as possible and seal the bag. Give the bag a good shake. It is now ready to freeze.

To Cook

1. Defrost the zip lock bag overnight in the fridge then empty the ingredients into a slow cooker.
2. Cook for 5–6 hours on LOW.
3. Adjust the seasoning and stir through the cashew nuts if not already added.

Serving Suggestion

Serve the cashew chicken over rice.

Storage & Reheating

Once this dish is cooked, leftovers will keep for 5–7 days in the fridge and 2–3 months in the freezer. Cooked meals can be frozen. Cool completely before chilling or freezing.

If cooking from frozen, defrost overnight in the fridge, then reheat the meal thoroughly in a microwave or saucepan.

Easy Asian Chicken & Rice Soup

Ingredients

300 g (approximately 1) chicken
    breast, sliced into 3 cm pieces

300g (approximately 2) chicken
    thighs, boneless, sliced into
    3 cm pieces

1 cup basmati rice

1 onion, chopped

2 carrots, diced

3 celery stalks, diced

4 garlic cloves, finely chopped

4 cm piece ginger, finely chopped

1 bunch coriander, stalks and
    roots finely chopped, leaves
    picked off

2 teaspoons light soy sauce

1 teaspoon brown sugar

½ teaspoon black pepper

2 tablespoons olive oil

1.5 litres chicken stock

Method

Place a zip lock bag in a large bowl and add all of the ingredients
(except the stock) to the bag. Squeeze out as much air as possible and
seal. Give the bag a good shake. It is now ready to freeze.

To Cook

1. Defrost the zip lock bag overnight in the fridge then empty the
   ingredients into a slow cooker.
2. Add 2 cups water and the stock then cook for 7–8 hours on LOW.
3. At the end of cooking, shred the chicken and return it to the soup.
   Season to taste and garnish with coriander leaves.

Storage & Reheating

Once this dish is cooked, leftovers will keep for 5–7 days in the fridge
and 2–3 months in the freezer. Cooked meals can be frozen. Cool
completely before chilling or freezing.

    If cooking from frozen, defrost overnight in the fridge, then reheat
the meal thoroughly in a microwave or saucepan.

Boston Beans

Ingredients

400 g dried cannellini or white
  beans, soaked overnight

1 onion, chopped

3 garlic cloves, finely chopped

5 rashers smoky bacon, thinly
  sliced

2 tablespoons smoked paprika

¼ cup brown sugar

¼ cup molasses

2 tablespoons cider vinegar

3 tablespoons tomato paste

½ teaspoon salt

½ teaspoon black pepper

Method

Drain the white beans and place in a zip lock bag along with the other ingredients. Squeeze out as much air as possible and seal the bag. Give the bag a good shake. It is now ready to freeze.

To Cook

1. Defrost the zip lock bag overnight in the fridge then empty the ingredients into a slow cooker along with 3 cups water.
2. Cook 6–7 hours on LOW.

Serving Suggestion

Serve the beans with crusty buttered bread on the side.

Storage & Reheating

Once this dish is cooked, leftovers will keep for 5–7 days in the fridge and 2–3 months in the freezer. Cooked meals can be frozen. Cool completely before chilling or freezing.

   If cooking from frozen, defrost overnight in the fridge, then reheat the meal thoroughly in a microwave or saucepan.

Slow Cooker Pork Pot Roast

You will need an extra-large zip lock bag for this meal.

Ingredients

2 teaspoons ground cumin
1 tablespoon smoked paprika
1 tablespoon salt
1 teaspoon black pepper
1.5 kg pork loin roast

1 onion, chopped
4 garlic cloves, finely chopped
4 carrots, cut into large dice
1 tablespoon olive oil

Method

1. Combine the cumin, paprika, salt and pepper in a small bowl, then rub all over the pork.
2. Place the zip lock bag in a large bowl and place the pork along with the remaining ingredients in the bag. Squeeze out as much air as possible and seal the bag. Give the bag a good shake. It is now ready to freeze.

To Cook

1. Defrost the zip lock bag overnight in the fridge then empty the ingredients into a slow cooker with 600 ml water.
2. Cook for 6–8 hours on LOW or until the meat is fall-apart tender.

Serving Suggestion

Serve with mashed potatoes and a green salad.

Storage & Reheating

Once this dish is cooked, leftovers will keep for 5–7 days in the fridge and 2–3 months in the freezer. Cooked meals can be frozen. Cool completely before chilling or freezing.

If cooking from frozen, defrost overnight in the fridge. Reheat thoroughly in a baking dish with a little water in a moderate oven (180°C) for approximately 30–40 minutes or until heated through.

Short-Cut Jambalaya

Ingredients

500 g chicken thighs, boneless, diced into 2-cm cubes

3 smoked sausages (chorizo or similar), thinly sliced

1 onion, chopped

1 green capsicum, diced

3 celery stalks, diced

4 garlic cloves, finely chopped

2 x 400 g tins whole peeled tomatoes

2 cups chicken stock

½ teaspoon cayenne pepper

1 teaspoon smoked paprika

1 teaspoon dried oregano

1½ cups long-grain rice

1 bunch parsley, leaves finely chopped, to garnish

Method

Place a zip lock bag in a large bowl and add all of the ingredients to the bag except the rice and parsley. Squeeze out as much air as possible and seal. Give the bag a good shake. It is now ready to freeze.

To Cook

1. Defrost the zip lock bag overnight in the fridge then empty the ingredients into a slow cooker.
2. Cook for 5 hours on LOW.
3. Stir in the rice and cook for a further 1 hour on LOW.
4. Garnish with parsley and serve.

Serving Suggestion

Serve on a bed of seasoned baby spinach.

Storage & Reheating

Once this dish is cooked, leftovers will keep for 5–7 days in the fridge and 2–3 months in the freezer. Cooked meals can be frozen. Cool completely before chilling or freezing.

If cooking from frozen, defrost overnight in the fridge, then reheat the meal thoroughly in a microwave or saucepan.

Coconut Chicken Curry

Ingredients

1 onion, roughly chopped

3 garlic cloves, roughly chopped

1 bunch coriander, stalks and roots washed and blended, leaves picked off

2 tablespoons tomato paste

1 x 400 ml tin coconut milk

1 teaspoon salt

1 tablespoon garam masala

1 tablespoon curry powder

500 g chicken breasts, diced into 3-cm cubes

500 g chicken thighs, boneless, diced into 3-cm cubes

2 sweet potatoes, peeled and diced into 3-cm cubes

1 red capsicum, cut into 1 cm-long strips

Method

1. Blend the onion, garlic, coriander stalks and roots, tomato paste, coconut milk, salt and spices in a food processor or blender.
2. Place a zip lock bag in a large bowl and place the curry paste and remaining ingredients in the bag. Squeeze out as much air as possible and seal. Give the bag a good shake. It is now ready to freeze.

To Cook

1. Defrost the zip lock bag overnight in the fridge then empty the ingredients into a slow cooker.
2. Add 4 tablespoons water and cook for 6–7 hours on LOW.
3. Adjust the seasoning, to taste. Serve garnished with the coriander leaves.

Serving Suggestion

Serve curry with basmati rice on the side.

Storage & Reheating

Once this dish is cooked, leftovers will keep for 5–7 days in the fridge and 2–3 months in the freezer. Cooked meals can be frozen. Cool completely before chilling or freezing.

If cooking from frozen, defrost overnight in the fridge, then reheat the meal thoroughly in a microwave or saucepan.

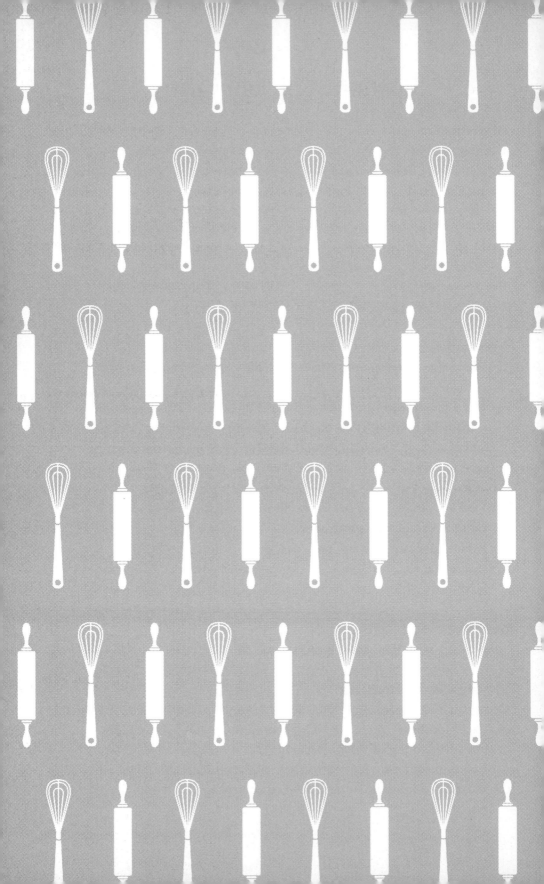

Meat & Veg Mix-Up! Slow Cooker Meals

Meat & Veg Mix-Up! Slow Cooker Meals

Mix up the menu this week, with some rich and hearty meat dishes, balanced with two nights of flavourful and nourishing vegetarian options. Each meal in this plan serves 6 people but if your family comprises 3–4 members, rather than reduce these recipes, use the leftovers for lunches and of course, freeze some for back-up meals!

The Slow Cooker Baggie Method

With our slow cooker plans you will notice there is not the usual Once-A-Week Cooking Plan section because we use our famed Baggie Method. This is where you pop all the meal ingredients into a large zip lock baggie, freeze it and then pull it out of the freezer when you're ready to cook it up.

You will find specific Baggie instructions underneath each individual recipe.

Here's how it works:

- Get 7 large zip lock baggies. Label each baggie with the name of the dish it will contain and the date of preparation. Also, add the cooking time and temperature that the slow cooker should be set to.
- Place each labelled baggie into one of 7 large bowls.
- Fill each labelled baggie with the ingredients as you prepare them. (For example, divide the chopped onions among baggies for dishes that contain chopped onion.)
- Refer to the recipes to see what other ingredients need to be added to each baggie before sealing and freezing.

Menu

Sausages with Onion & Capsicum

Mexican Chicken

Slow Cooker Friendly Meatballs

Red Lentil Soup

Chana Masala

Irish Beef Stew

Thai Peanut Chicken Drumsticks

Shopping List

Meat & Fish	Fruit & Veg	Dairy & Frozen
400 g pork sausages 700 g chicken breasts 1 kg chicken drumsticks 700 g beef mince 1 kg beef (chuck, bolar or oyster blade)	7 onions 2 heads garlic 1 x 8 cm piece ginger 5 potatoes 7 carrots 1 bunch celery 4 red capsicums 2 corn cobs 1 jalapeño chilli 1 large red chilli 1 bunch coriander 1 bunch Vietnamese mint 2 bunches basil 1 bunch thyme 1 lemon 1 lime	1 egg ⅓ cup milk 2 cups frozen peas

Tins, Jars & Dry Goods	Pantry Essentials	Other Ingredients
5 x 400 g tins whole peeled tomatoes 2 x 400 g tins crushed tomatoes 2 cups dry chickpeas 1 cup dry black beans 2 cups red lentils ⅓ cup breadcrumbs	canola, sunflower or grapeseed oil 1.25 litres chicken stock 1.25 litres vegetable stock 1 jar tomato paste ½ cup flour ¼ cup plus 1 tbs brown sugar salt pepper 3 tbs soy sauce 3 tbs sweet chilli sauce ⅓ cup peanut or almond butter 5 tsp smoked paprika 5 tsp ground cumin 2 tbs plus 1 tsp ground coriander 2 tsp garam masala 1 tsp turmeric	1 cup Guinness or other stout 10–12 soft flour or corn tortillas

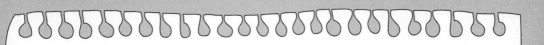

Serving Size
Each meal serves a family of 4–6

Preparation time
1 hour

Equipment
Slow cooker (minimum 5-litre), sharp knives, chopping boards suitable for vegetables and fruit, meat and fish, kitchen scales, measuring cups and spoons, vegetable peeler, food processor, baking trays, large mixing bowls, large zip lock bags.

Storage & Reheating
While you can generally keep meat and vegetables in the fridge for the week, because these meals have combined ingredients, it is necessary to freeze them straightaway. You can keep the meal you plan to cook the next day and the day after in the fridge, but the rest should be frozen. This is due to the potential for cross-contamination of germs or bacteria. Once ingredients are combined, the environment becomes more suitable for growing bacteria, so freezing or cooking is necessary.

Defrost each meal overnight then put in the slow cooker the day you plan to eat it. Avoid defrosting meals and leaving them without cooking for a full day and night.

Once each dish is cooked, leftovers will keep for 5–7 days in the fridge. Once cooked, the meals can be frozen. Just make sure that you defrost and reheat the meal very thoroughly.

Once-A-Week Cooking Preparation

	Total	Sausages with Onion & Capsicum	Mexican Chicken	Slow Cooker Friendly Meatballs
Dry goods				
Black beans (cups)	1		1 cup, soaked in cold water overnight	
Chickpeas (cups)	2			
Fresh Produce				
Onions	7	1, thinly sliced	1 thinly sliced	1 finely chopped
Garlic heads	1	2 cloves, thinly sliced	4 cloves, thinly sliced	2 cloves, finely chopped
Ginger	8 cm piece			
Potatoes	7			
Carrots	7			
Celery	1			
Capsicums	4	3 red, julienned	1 red, sliced	
Corn	2		2 cobs, kernels stripped	
Jalapeño chilli	1		1 thinly sliced	
Red chilli	1			
Coriander	1		1 bunch, stalks and roots finely chopped, leaves finely chopped	
Basil	2			1 bunch, finely chopped
Thyme	1			
Lemon	1			
Lime	1		1 juiced	
Vietnamese mint	1			
Meat				
Pork sausages	400 g	diagonally cut into 1 cm-thick pieces		
Chicken breasts	700 g		butterflied	
Beef chuck, bolar or oyster blade	1 kg			

Red Lentil Soup	Chana Masala	Irish Beef Stew	Thai Peanut Chicken Drumsticks
	2 cups, soaked in cold water overnight		
1 chopped	2 finely chopped	1 chopped	
3 cloves, finely chopped	3 cloves, finely chopped	4 cloves, finely chopped	2 cloves, finely chopped
	4 cm piece, finely chopped		4 cm piece, finely chopped
		5 quartered	
3 diced		4 diced	
3 stalks, diced		4 stalks, diced	
	1 thinly sliced		
1 bunch, finely chopped			
5 sprigs, leaves picked			
	1 juiced		
			1 bunch, finely chopped
		diced into 3-cm cubes	

Sausages with Onion & Capsicum

Ingredients

400 g good-quality pork sausages, diagonally cut into 1 cm-thick pieces

1 onion, thinly sliced

2 garlic cloves, thinly sliced

3 red capsicums, julienned

2 x 400 g tins whole peeled tomatoes

½ cup chicken stock

2 teaspoons smoked paprika

½ teaspoon salt

½ teaspoon pepper

Method

Place a zip lock bag in a large bowl and add all of the ingredients to the bowl. Squeeze out as much air as possible and seal. Give the bag a good shake. It is now ready to freeze.

To Cook

1. Defrost the zip lock bag overnight in the fridge then empty the ingredients into a slow cooker.
2. Cook for 6 hours on HIGH.

Serving Suggestion

Serve with steamed brown rice on the side.

Storage & Reheating

This dish will keep for 3–4 days in the fridge and 2–3 months in the freezer. Once cooked, cool completely before chilling or freezing.

If cooking from frozen, defrost overnight in the fridge, then reheat the meal thoroughly in a microwave or saucepan.

Mexican Chicken

Ingredients

1 cup black beans, soaked in cold water overnight

700 g chicken breasts, butterflied

1 onion, thinly sliced

4 garlic cloves, finely chopped

1 red capsicum, sliced

2 corn cobs, kernels stripped

1 jalapeño chilli, thinly sliced

1 bunch coriander, stems and roots finely chopped, leaves finely chopped, for garnish

2 teaspoons cumin

1 teaspoon smoked paprika

½ teaspoon salt

½ teaspoon pepper

juice of 1 lime, for garnish

10–12 soft flour or corn tortillas

Method

Drain the beans and place in a zip lock bag. Add the remaining ingredients except the coriander leaves and lime juice. Squeeze out as much air as possible and seal. Give the bag a good shake. It is now ready to freeze.

To Cook

1. Defrost the zip lock bag overnight in the fridge then empty the ingredients into a slow cooker.
2. Cook for 7–8 hours on LOW.
3. Warm tortillas in the oven then stuff with the chicken and bean mixture. Garnish with coriander leaves and lime juice.

Serving Suggestion

Serve with a green salad, sour cream and lime wedges.

Storage & Reheating

Cooked chicken will keep for up to 4 days in the fridge and 1–2 months in the freezer. Cool completely before chilling or freezing.

If cooking from frozen, defrost overnight in the fridge, then reheat the meal thoroughly in a microwave or saucepan.

Slow Cooker Friendly Meatballs

Ingredients

Meatballs

⅓ cup breadcrumbs or 2 slices
 white bread, torn
⅓ cup milk
700 g beef mince
1 onion, finely chopped

2 garlic cloves, finely chopped
1 egg
1 teaspoon salt
½ teaspoon pepper

Sauce

2 x 400 g tins whole peeled
 tomatoes
1 tablespoon brown sugar

1 teaspoon salt
½ teaspoon pepper
1 bunch basil, finely chopped

Method

1. Soak the breadcrumbs or torn white bread in the milk for a
   few minutes.
2. In a large bowl, combine all of the meatball ingredients and roll into
   balls about 3 cm across. Place on a lined baking tray and freeze.
3. Once frozen, place the meatballs in a large zip lock bag and the
   ingredients for the sauce in a separate zip lock bag. Return the
   meatballs to the freezer and place the sauce in the fridge, as it needs
   to be liquid before adding to a slow cooker.

To Cook

1. Do not defrost the meatballs. Place in a slow cooker with the sauce.
2. Cook for 6–7 hours on LOW.

Serving Suggestion

Serve on top of cooked pasta and parmesan shavings.

Storage & Reheating

Cooked meatballs in sauce will keep for 3–4 days in the fridge and 2–3 months in the freezer. Cool completely before chilling or freezing.

If cooking from frozen, defrost overnight in the fridge, then reheat the meal thoroughly in a microwave or saucepan.

Red Lentil Soup

Ingredients

2 cups red lentils, rinsed
1 onion, chopped
3 garlic cloves, finely chopped
3 carrots, diced
3 celery stalks, diced
3 tablespoons tomato paste
1 bunch basil, leaves finely
    chopped

5 thyme sprigs, leaves picked
1 teaspoon ground coriander
1 teaspoon ground cumin
1 teaspoon salt
½ teaspoon black pepper
1 x 400 g tin whole peeled
    tomatoes
1 litre vegetable stock

Method

Place a zip lock bag in a bowl and add all of the ingredients. If you
need to save freezer space, you can leave out the tinned tomatoes and
vegetable stock and add these the morning of the day you plan to cook
the soup. Squeeze out as much air as possible and seal. Give the bag a
good shake. It is now ready to freeze.

To Cook

1. Defrost the zip lock bag overnight in the fridge then empty the
    ingredients into a slow cooker.
2. Cook for 8–10 hours on LOW.

Serving Suggestion

Serve soup with buttered crusty bread (and dunk!).

Storage & Reheating

The soup will keep for up to 1 week in the fridge and 2–3 months in
the freezer. If freezing, store the soup in portion-sized containers. Cool
completely before chilling or freezing.

  If cooking from frozen, defrost overnight in the fridge, then reheat
the meal thoroughly in a microwave or saucepan.

Chana Masala

MamaBaker Natalie loves this dish and shares her memory of when she first discovered it:

"Chana Masala is a beautiful North Indian dish I first enjoyed when I was travelling in the foothills of the Himalayas. It is made with chickpeas and aromatic spices. It is a wholesome warming dish for everyone in the family, and superb if you're on a tight budget."

Ingredients

2 cups chickpeas, soaked in cold
  water overnight
2 onions, finely chopped
3 cloves garlic, finely chopped
4 cm piece ginger, finely chopped
1 large red chilli, thinly sliced
1 tablespoon ground coriander
2 teaspoons cumin
2 teaspoons smoked paprika

2 teaspoons garam masala
1 teaspoon turmeric
2 x 400 g tins crushed tomatoes
1 cup vegetable stock
1 tablespoon oil
1 teaspoon salt
½ teaspoon pepper
juice of 1 lemon

Method

Drain the chickpeas and place in a zip lock bag along with the remaining ingredients except the lemon juice. Squeeze out as much air as possible and seal. Give the bag a good shake. It is now ready to freeze.

To Cook

1. Defrost the zip lock bag overnight in the fridge then empty the ingredients into a slow cooker.
2. Cook for 5–6 hours on LOW.
3. Squeeze in the lemon juice and give everything a good stir.

Serving Suggestion

Serve the Chana Masala with steamed basmati rice on the side.

Storage & Reheating

This dish will keep for up to 1 week in the fridge and 2–3 months in the freezer. Once cooked, allow to cool completely before chilling or freezing.

If cooking from frozen, defrost overnight in the fridge, then reheat the meal thoroughly in a microwave or saucepan.

Irish Beef Stew

Ingredients

½ cup flour

2 teaspoons salt

½ teaspoon pepper

1 kg beef chuck, bolar or oyster
blade, diced into 3-cm cubes

1 onion, chopped

4 garlic cloves, finely chopped

4 carrots, diced

4 celery sticks, diced

5 medium potatoes, quartered

1 litre chicken stock

1 cup Guinness or other stout

4 tablespoons tomato paste

2 cups frozen peas

Method

1. Place the flour, salt and pepper in a large zip lock bag. Add the meat, seal the bag and give it a good shake to coat the meat.
2. Add the remaining ingredients except the peas. Squeeze out as much air as possible and seal. Give the bag a good shake. It is now ready to freeze.

To Cook

1. Defrost the zip lock bag overnight in the fridge then empty the ingredients into a slow cooker.
2. Cook for 7–8 hours on LOW.
3. In the last 10 minutes of cooking add the frozen peas and stir through.

Serving Suggestion

Serve with crusty bread to mop up the juices.

Storage & Reheating

The cooked stew will keep for 5 days in the fridge. Cooked meals can be frozen for up to 2–3 months. Cool completely before chilling or freezing.

If cooking from frozen, defrost overnight in the fridge, then reheat the meal thoroughly in a microwave or saucepan.

Thai Peanut Chicken Drumsticks

Ingredients

1 kg chicken drumsticks

4 cm piece of ginger, finely
chopped

2 garlic cloves, finely chopped

⅓ cup peanut or almond butter

3 tablespoons soy sauce

3 tablespoons sweet chilli sauce

¼ cup brown sugar

1 tablespoon ground coriander

1 bunch Vietnamese mint, finely
chopped, for garnish

Method

Place a zip lock bag in a large bowl and add all the ingredients to the
bag, except the Vietnamese mint. Squeeze out as much air as possible
and seal. Give the bag a good shake. It is now ready to freeze.

To Cook

1. Defrost the zip lock bag overnight in the fridge then empty the
   ingredients into a slow cooker.
2. Cook for 6–8 hours on LOW.
3. Garnish with the Vietnamese mint and serve.

Serving Suggestion

Serve the chicken drumsticks with steamed basmati rice and green salad
leaves on the side, with lime wedges for squeezing over.

Storage & Reheating

The cooked chicken will keep for up to 4 days in the fridge or
2 months in the freezer. Once cooked, allow to cool completely
before chilling or freezing.

   If cooking from frozen, defrost overnight in the fridge, then
reheat the meal thoroughly in a microwave or saucepan.

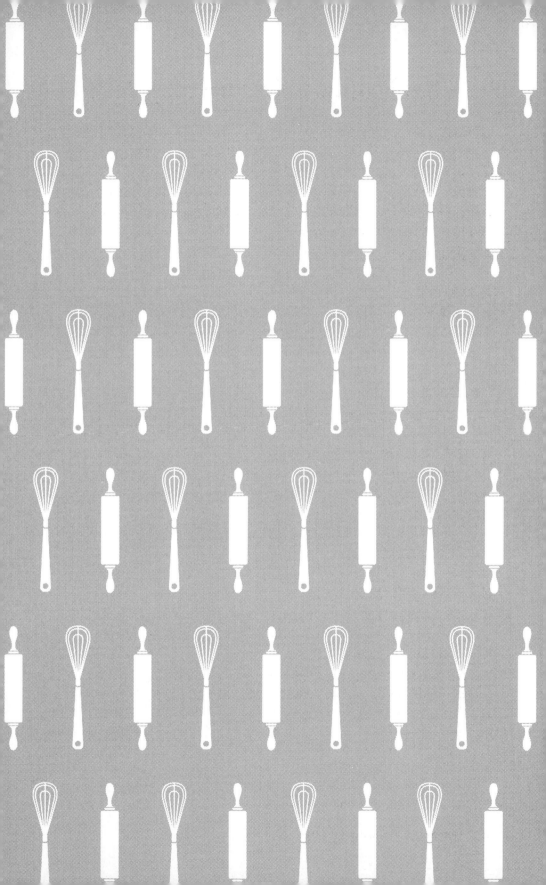

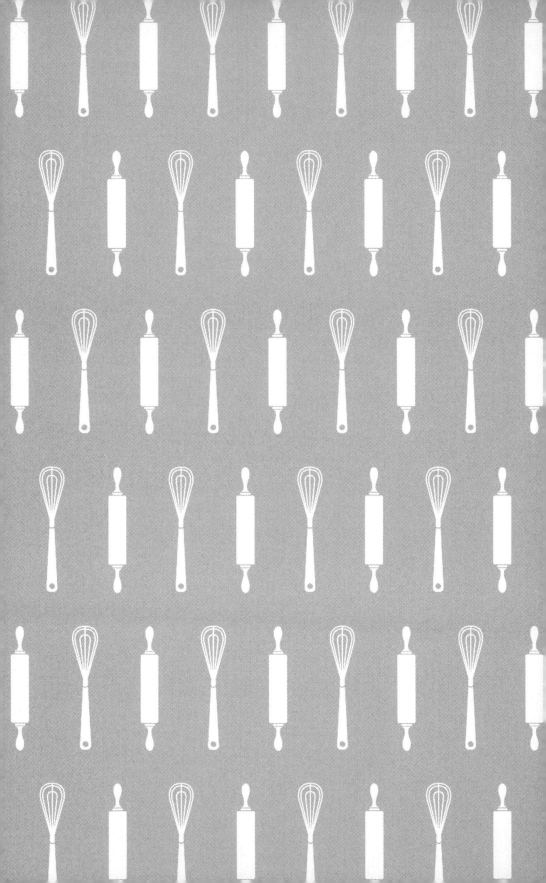

The Slow Cooker Mid-Week Dinner Party Plan

━━ The Slow Cooker ━━ Mid-Week Dinner Party Plan

This plan includes a real centrepiece dish: Cassoulet, a rich French stew combining various cuts of pork and beans. It is absolutely delicious on a cold day and is wonderful for a long weekend lunch or dinner with friends. Choose any of the seven recipes in this plan and host a mid-week dinner party with friends.

The Slow Cooker Baggie Method

With our slow cooker plans you will notice there is not the usual Once-A-Week Cooking Plan section because we use our famed Baggie Method. This is where you pop all the meal ingredients into a large zip lock baggie, freeze it and then pull it out of the freezer when you're ready to cook it up.

You will find specific Baggie instructions underneath each individual recipe.

Here's how it works:

- Get 7 large zip lock baggies. Label each baggie with the name of the dish it will contain and the date of preparation. Also, add the cooking time and temperature that the slow cooker should be set to.
- Place each labelled baggie into one of 7 large bowls.
- Fill each labelled baggie with the ingredients as you prepare them. (For example, divide the chopped onions among baggies for dishes that contain chopped onion.)
- Refer to the recipes to see what other ingredients need to be added to each baggie before sealing and freezing.

Menu

Slow Cooker Cassoulet

Vegetable Soup

Cuban-Style Shredded Pork

Sweet & Sour Chicken

Beef & Barley Stew

Thai Peanut Pork

Pumpkin, Cranberry & Pecan Rice

Shopping List

Meat & Fish	Fruit & Veg	Dairy & Frozen
500 g chicken thighs, boneless 900 g chicken breasts 500 g beef chuck steak 3 kg pork shoulder, boneless 500 g pork sausages	5 onions 2 heads garlic 1 x 4 cm piece ginger 12 carrots 1 leek 1 butternut pumpkin 1 bunch celery 1 red chilli 3 red capsicums 3 spring onions 3 handfuls baby spinach 1 bunch rosemary 1 bunch thyme 1 bunch oregano 1 bunch dill 1 lime	none

Tins, Jars & Dry Goods	Pantry Essentials	Other Ingredients
5 x 400 g tins whole peeled tomatoes 1 x 400 g tin pineapple in juice 2 cups dried cannellini beans 2 x 400 g tins cooked cannellini beans 1 cup puy lentils ½ cup pearl barley 4 cups long-grain rice ½ cup dried cranberries 1 cup pecans	olive oil 2.25 litres chicken stock 2.75 litres vegetable stock 2 tbs tomato paste 2 tbs white vinegar salt pepper ⅓ cup peanut or almond butter ½ cup peanut butter ½ cup plus 2 tbs soy sauce 3 tbs honey ⅓ cup tomato sauce (ketchup) 2 tsp ground coriander 2 tsp ground cumin 2 tsp dried oregano 1 bay leaf	1 cup white or red wine

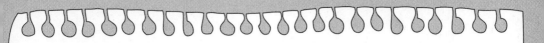

Serving Size

Each meal serves 4–6 people

Preparation time

1½ hours

Equipment

Slow cooker (minimum 5-litre), sharp knives, chopping boards suitable for vegetables and fruit, meat and fish, kitchen scales, measuring cups and spoons, vegetable peeler, large mixing bowls and large zip lock bags.

Storage & Reheating

While you can generally keep meat and vegetables in the fridge for the week, because these meals have combined ingredients, it is necessary to freeze them straightaway. You can keep the meal you plan to cook the next day and the day after in the fridge, but the rest should be frozen. Defrost each meal overnight then put in the slow cooker the day you plan to eat it. Avoid defrosting meals and leaving them without cooking for a full day and night.

Once each dish is cooked, leftovers will keep for 5–7 days in the fridge. Once cooked, the meals can be frozen. Just make sure that you defrost and reheat the meal very thoroughly.

Once-A-Week Cooking Preparation

	Total	Slow Cooker Cassoulet	Vegetable Soup	Cuban-Style Shredded Pork
Dry goods				
Cannellini beans		2 cups soaked in cold water overnight	1 cup soaked in cold water overnight	
Pecans				
Fresh Produce				
Onions	5	1 chopped	1 finely chopped	1 quartered
Garlic	2	3 cloves, finely chopped	4 cloves, finely chopped	6 cloves, finely chopped
Ginger	4 cm piece			
Carrots	12	3 diced	3 finely diced	
Leek	1		1 finely diced	
Butternut pumpkin	1			
Celery	1		3 stalks, finely diced	
Red capsicums	3			
Rosemary	1	3 sprigs, leaves picked		
Thyme	1	3 sprigs, leaves picked	3 sprigs, leaves picked	
Oregano	1		5 sprigs, leaves picked	
Dill	1			
Red chilli	1			
Spring onions	3			
Lime	1			juiced
Meat				
Chicken thighs, boneless	500 g	500 g, each thigh quartered		
Chicken breasts	900 g			
Beef chuck steak	500 g			
Pork shoulder	3 kg	reserve 400 g and dice into 2-cm cubes		reserve 1.8 kg and cut into 4 pieces
Pork Sausages	500 g	500 g cut in half crossways		

Sweet & Sour Chicken	Beef & Barley Stew	Thai Peanut Pork	Pumpkin, Cranberry & Pecan Rice
			1 cup, toasted
1 chopped	1 chopped		
3 cloves, finely chopped	3 cloves, finely chopped	2 cloves, finely chopped	3 cloves, finely chopped
		finely chopped	
2 cut into 6–8 pieces	4 diced		
			peeled, seeds removed, flesh cut into 5-cm chunks
	3 stalks diced		
1 cut into large dice		2 cut into large dice	
	3 sprigs, leaves picked		
	3 sprigs, leaves picked		4 sprigs, leaves picked
			1 bunch, finely chopped
		1 finely chopped	
3 thinly sliced			
each breast cut into 8 pieces			
	cut into 3-cm pieces		
		reserve 800 g and dice into 2-cm cubes	

Slow Cooker Cassoulet

Ingredients

2 cups cannellini beans, soaked in cold water overnight

500 g chicken thighs, boneless, quartered

400 g boneless pork shoulder, diced into 2-cm cubes

500 g pork sausages, cut in half crossways

1 onion, chopped

3 carrots, diced

3 garlic cloves, finely chopped

3 rosemary sprigs, leaves picked

3 thyme sprigs, leaves picked

2 x 400 g tins whole peeled tomatoes

2 tablespoons tomato paste

2 cups chicken stock

1 cup white or red wine

½ teaspoon salt

½ teaspoon pepper

Method

Drain the cannellini beans and place in a zip lock bag with the remaining ingredients. Squeeze out as much air as possible and seal. Give the bag a good shake. It is now ready to freeze.

To Cook

1. Defrost the zip lock bag overnight in the fridge then empty the ingredients into a slow cooker.
2. Cook for 7–8 hours on LOW.

Serving Suggestion

Serve the cassoulet with crusty bread on the side.

Storage & Reheating

This dish will keep for 3–4 days in the fridge and 2–3 months in the freezer. Once cooked, cool completely before chilling or freezing.

If cooking from frozen, defrost overnight in the fridge, then follow steps 1 and 2 to cook.

Vegetable Soup

Ingredients

1 onion, finely chopped

1 leek, finely diced

4 garlic cloves, finely chopped

3 carrots, finely diced

3 celery stalks, finely diced

5 oregano sprigs, leaves picked

3 thyme sprigs, leaves picked and stalks discarded

1 tablespoon olive oil

1 cup long-grain rice

½ teaspoon salt

½ teaspoon pepper

3 x 400 g tins whole peeled tomatoes

1.5 litres vegetable stock

2 x 400 g tins cooked cannellini beans

Method

Place all the ingredients except for the cannellini beans in a zip lock bag. If you need to save freezer space, you can omit the tinned tomatoes and vegetable stock and add these the morning of the day you plan to cook the soup. Squeeze out as much air as possible and seal. Give the bag a good shake. It is now ready to freeze.

To Cook

1. Defrost the zip lock bag overnight in the fridge then empty the ingredients into a slow cooker.
2. Cook for 4–6 hours on LOW.
3. Add the cannellini beans to the slow cooker 15 minutes before the end of cooking.

Serving Suggestion

Serve steaming with crusty bread rolls.

Storage & Reheating

Once cooked, the soup will keep for up to 1 week in the fridge. Cool completely before chilling or freezing.

This soup can be frozen for up to 3 months.

If cooking from frozen, defrost overnight in the fridge, then reheat the meal thoroughly in a microwave or saucepan.

Cuban-Style Shredded Pork

Ingredients

6 garlic cloves, finely chopped

2 teaspoons ground cumin

2 teaspoons ground coriander

2 teaspoons dried oregano

1½ teaspoons salt

½ teaspoon pepper

1.8 kg boneless pork shoulder, cut into 4 pieces

1 onion, quartered

juice of 1 lime

Method

Combine the garlic, spices, salt and pepper in a small bowl. Rub the spice mix all over the pork. Place the pork, onion, lime juice and 1 cup water in a zip lock bag. Squeeze out as much air as possible and seal. Give the bag a good shake. It is now ready to freeze.

To Cook

1. Defrost the zip lock bag overnight in the fridge then empty the ingredients into a slow cooker.
2. Cook for 8 hours on LOW. When cooked, use two forks to shred the cooked pork.

Serving Suggestion

Serve on soft bread rolls with sour cream and salad greens.

Storage & Reheating

The shredded pork will keep for up to one week in the fridge or 1–2 months in the freezer. Cool completely before chilling or freezing.

If cooking from frozen, defrost overnight in the fridge then reheat the meat thoroughly in a microwave or toss in a hot frying pan for chewy, crispy pork.

Sweet & Sour Chicken

Ingredients

900 g chicken breasts, each breast cut into 8 pieces

1 onion, chopped

3 garlic cloves, finely chopped

2 carrots, each cut into 6–8 pieces

1 red capsicum, chopped into large dice

1 x 400 g tin pineapple in juice

⅓ cup tomato sauce (ketchup) (the secret to this dish)

2 tablespoons soy sauce

2 tablespoons white vinegar

2 cups chicken stock

3 spring onions, thinly sliced

Method

Place a zip lock bag in a bowl and add all of the ingredients to the bag except the spring onion. Squeeze out as much air as possible and seal. Give the bag a good shake. It is now ready to freeze.

To Cook

1. Defrost the zip lock bag overnight in the fridge then empty the ingredients into a slow cooker.
2. Cook for 6–8 hours on LOW.
3. Garnish with the spring onion.

Serving Suggestion

Serve with steamed basmati rice on the side.

Storage & Reheating

This dish will keep for 3–4 days in the fridge and up to 2 months in the freezer. Cool completely before chilling or freezing.

If cooking from frozen, defrost overnight in the fridge. Reheat the meal thoroughly in a microwave or saucepan.

Beef & Barley Stew

Ingredients

500 g beef chuck steak, cut into
    3 cm pieces
1 onion, chopped
3 garlic cloves, finely chopped
4 carrots, diced
3 celery stalks, diced
3 thyme sprigs, leaves picked

3 rosemary sprigs, leaves picked
1 bay leaf
1 teaspoon salt
¼ teaspoon pepper
¼ cup pearl barley
1 litre chicken stock

Method

Place a large zip lock bag in a bowl and add all the ingredients except
the chicken stock to the bag. Squeeze out as much air as possible and
seal. Give the bag a good shake. It is now ready to freeze.

To Cook

1. Defrost the zip lock bag overnight in the fridge then empty the
   ingredients into a slow cooker along with the chicken stock and
   5 cups water.
2. Cook for 8 hours on LOW.
3. Remove the bay leaf and serve.

Serving Suggestion

Warmed crusty bread with lashings of butter to mop up the gravy.

Storage & Reheating

The cooked stew will keep for 4 days in the fridge or 2–3 months in the
freezer. Cool completely before chilling and freezing.

    If cooking from frozen, defrost overnight in the fridge. Reheat the
meal thoroughly in a microwave or saucepan.

Thai Peanut Pork

Ingredients

800 g boneless pork shoulder,
   diced into 2 cm cubes

4 cm piece ginger, finely chopped

1 mild red chilli, thinly sliced

2 garlic cloves, finely chopped

2 red capsicums, chopped into
   large dice

½ cup peanut butter

½ cup soy sauce

3 tablespoons honey

1 cup chicken stock

Method

Place a large zip lock bag in a bowl and add all of the ingredients to the bag. Squeeze out as much air as possible and seal. Give the bag a good shake. It is now ready to freeze.

To Cook

1. Defrost the zip lock bag overnight in the fridge then empty the ingredients into a slow cooker.
2. Cook for 5 hours on LOW. Then, remove the lid and cook for an additional 1 hour. Alternatively cook for 6 hours on low and then remove the meat and vegetables from the sauce. Reduce the sauce by one-third in a separate saucepan.

Serving Suggestion

Serve with steamed rice.

Storage & Reheating

This dish will keep for up to 4 days in the fridge and up to 2 months in the freezer. Cool completely before chilling or freezing.

If cooking from frozen, defrost overnight in the fridge. Reheat the meal thoroughly in a microwave or saucepan. Alternatively, fry for extra crispness.

Pumpkin, Cranberry & Pecan Rice

Ingredients

1 cup puy lentils, rinsed

½ cup dried cranberries

1 cup pecans, toasted

3 garlic cloves, finely chopped

1 butternut pumpkin, peeled, seeds removed, flesh cut into 5 cm chunks

4 thyme sprigs, leaves picked

2 tablespoons olive oil

1 teaspoon salt

½ teaspoon pepper

1.25 litres vegetable stock

3 cups long-grain rice

3 handfuls baby spinach

1 bunch dill, finely chopped

Method

Place the zip lock bag in a large bowl and add the lentils, cranberries, pecans, garlic, pumpkin, thyme, oil and seasoning to the bag. Squeeze out as much air as possible and seal. Give the bag a good shake. It is now ready to freeze.

To Cook

1. There is no need to defrost the ingredients. Simply empty the ingredients into a slow cooker along with the vegetable stock.
2. Cook on LOW for 5 hours.
3. Add the rice and cook for a further 30 minutes.
4. Add the baby spinach and fresh dill for the last 5 minutes of cooking and stir through.

Storage & Reheating

This dish will keep for up to 3 days in the fridge. Once cooked, cool completely before chilling or freezing. It will keep in the freezer for up to 1 month.

If cooking from frozen, defrost overnight in the fridge. Reheat the meal thoroughly in a microwave or saucepan.

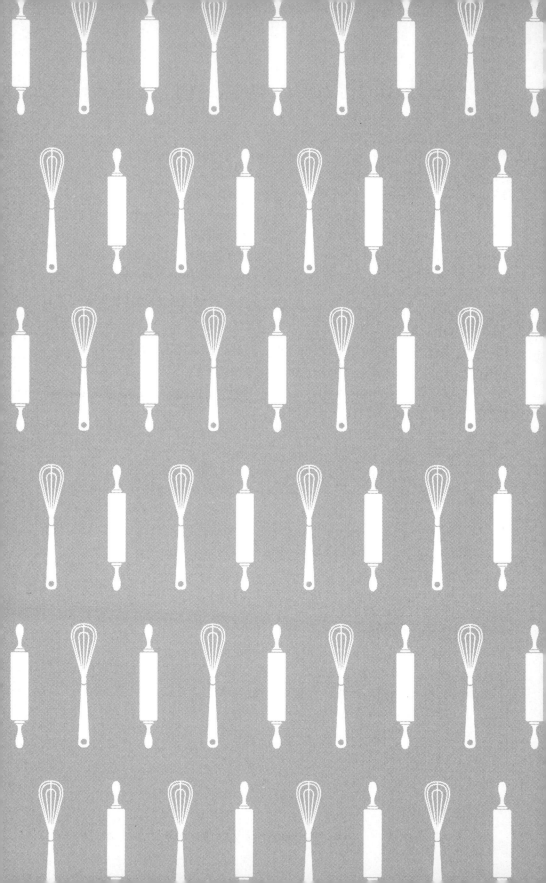

The Vegan Slow Cooker Menu

The Vegan Slow Cooker Menu

Here are some absolutely delicious vegan meals you can prepare for the week ahead. They are wholesome and full of flavour.

All of the ingredients listed in this plan can be frozen; however, if you need to save room in the freezer or your zip lock bag isn't quite big enough, you can simply leave out the tinned ingredients or items such as liquid stock and add them when you start cooking.

The Slow Cooker Baggie Method

With our slow cooker plans you will notice there is not the usual Once-A-Week Cooking Plan section because we use our famed Baggie Method. This is where you pop all the meal ingredients into a large zip lock baggie, freeze it and then pull it out of the freezer when you're ready to cook it up.

You will find specific Baggie instructions underneath each individual recipe.

Here's how it works:

- Get 7 large zip lock baggies. Label each baggie with the name of the dish it will contain and the date of preparation. Also, add the cooking time and temperature that the slow cooker should be set to.
- Place each labelled baggie into one of 7 large bowls.
- Fill each labelled baggie with the ingredients as you prepare them. (For example, divide the chopped onions among baggies for dishes that contain chopped onion.)
- Refer to the recipes to see what other ingredients need to be added to each baggie before sealing and freezing.

Menu

Chickpea Cauliflower Curry
with Coconut Rice

White Bean Stew

'Butter' Chickpeas & Tofu

Vegan Bolognese

Black Beans & Rice

Sweet Potato, Pumpkin, Carrot
& Split-Pea Soup

Indian Curried Eggplant

Shopping List

Meat & Fish	Fruit & Veg	Dairy & Frozen
none	7 onions 2 heads garlic 1 x 12 cm piece ginger 7 carrots 3 sweet potatoes 1½ butternut pumpkins 1 cauliflower 1 bunch celery 1 red capsicum 3 large eggplants 10 button mushrooms 1 medium green chilli 1 bunch spinach 1 bunch chard or kale 1 bunch rosemary 1 bunch thyme 2 bunches coriander 1 bunch basil 1 bunch oregano	none

Tins, Jars & Dry Goods	Pantry Essentials	Other Ingredients
7 x 400 g tins whole peeled tomatoes 1 x 400 g tin crushed tomatoes 3 x 200 ml tins coconut milk 2 cups dried chickpeas (or, 1½ x 400 g tinned chickpeas) 1 cup dried chickpeas 1 cup dried black beans 2 cups dried white beans ½ cup split peas 1 cup raw cashews 2 cups basmati rice 1 cup long-grain rice	canola, sunflower or grapeseed oil olive oil 3 litres vegetable stock 2 tbs tomato paste 2 tbs brown sugar salt pepper ⅓ cup peanut or almond butter 1 tsp sweet paprika 4 tsp ground cumin 1 tbs plus 1 tsp ground coriander 2 tsp chilli powder 2 tbs garam masala 2 tsp turmeric 1 tbs plus 2 tsp curry powder 1 tsp ground cardamom	400 g firm tofu

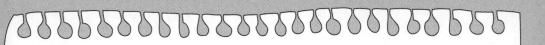

Serving Size
Each meal serves a family of 4–6

Preparation time
1 hour

Equipment
Slow cooker (minimum 5-litre), sharp knives, chopping board, kitchen scales, measuring cups and spoons, food processor, vegetable peeler, large mixing bowls and large zip lock bags.

Storage & Reheating
All prepped meals can be frozen or kept in the fridge for up to one week. If you are uncertain as to whether you will or will not eat these meals when you plan to, freeze them to be safe. They require no defrosting – just put the contents straight into the slow cooker.

Once cooked, each dish will keep for 5–7 days in the fridge. Alternatively, they can be frozen for 2–3 months but must be reheated very well.

The only dish that does not freeze well is the 'Butter' Chickpeas & Tofu, so you should consider eating this meal within a day or two of it being cooked.

Once-A-Week Cooking Preparation

	Total	Chickpea Cauliflower Curry with Coconut Rice	White Bean Stew	'Butter' Chickpeas & Tofu
Dry goods				
Chickpeas	3	2 cups, soaked in cold water overnight		1 cup, soaked in cold water overnight
Black beans	1			
White beans	2		2 cups, soaked in cold water overnight	
Fresh Produce				
Onions	7	1 chopped	1 chopped	1 chopped
Garlic heads	2	2 cloves, finely chopped	3 cloves, finely chopped	4 cloves, finely chopped
Ginger	12 cm piece	4 cm piece, finely chopped		4 cm piece, finely chopped
Carrots	7		1 diced	
Sweet potatoes	3	1 peeled and cut into large chunks		
Butternut pumpkin	1½			
Cauliflower	1	½ head, cut into florets		
Celery	1		3 stalks, diced	
Capsicum	1			
Eggplant	3			
Mushrooms	10			
Medium green chilli	1			
Chard or kale	1		1 bunch, stalks removed and leaves roughly chopped	
Spinach	1		1 bunch, stalks removed and leaves roughly chopped	
Coriander	2			1 bunch, stalks and roots finely chopped, leaves roughly chopped
Thyme	1		3 sprigs, leaves picked	
Rosemary	1		3 sprigs, leaves picked	
Basil	1			
Oregano	1			

Vegan Bolognese	Black Beans & Rice	Sweet Potato, Pumpkin, Carrot & Split-Pea Soup	Indian Curried Eggplant
	1 cup, soaked in cold water overnight		
1 chopped	1 finely chopped	1 chopped	1 chopped
4 cloves, chopped	3 cloves, finely chopped		3 cloves, finely chopped
			4 cm piece, finely chopped
3 grated		3 cut into large chunks	
		2 peeled and cut into large chunks	
½ peeled, seeds removed and flesh grated		1 peeled, seeds removed and flesh cut into chunks	
½ head, chopped			
3 stalks, diced			
	1 finely diced		
1 diced			2 chopped into 10–12 pieces each and soaked in water
10 diced			
			1 finely chopped
			1 bunch, stalks and roots finely chopped, leaves roughly chopped
		3 sprigs, leaves picked	
1 bunch, upper stalks finely chopped, leaves picked			
4 sprigs, leaves picked			

Chickpea Cauliflower Curry
with Coconut Rice

Ingredients

2 cups dried chickpeas, soaked in cold water overnight (or 1½ x 400 g tinned chickpeas)

1 tablespoon oil

1 onion, chopped

2 garlic cloves, finely chopped

4 cm piece ginger, finely chopped

1 tablespoon garam masala

1 teaspoon curry powder

½ cauliflower head, cut into florets

1 sweet potato, peeled and cut into large chunks

1 teaspoon salt

2 x 400 g tins whole peeled tomatoes

1 x 200 ml tin coconut milk

1 cup vegetable stock

Coconut Rice

2 cups basmati rice

1 x 200 ml tin coconut milk

¼ teaspoon salt

Method

1. Drain the chickpeas and set aside.
2. Heat the oil in a frying pan over medium heat. Sauté the onion, garlic and ginger until the onion is translucent. Add the spices and toast for a couple of minutes until fragrant. Set the mixture aside to cool. (Alternatively, you can skip this step and just put all of the ingredients in a zip lock bag, but toasting really boosts the flavour.)
3. Place a zip lock bag in a bowl and add all of the ingredients to the bag. If you need to save freezer space or your zip lock bag isn't quite big enough, simply leave out the tinned tomatoes, coconut milk and vegetable stock and add them when you start cooking. Squeeze out as much air as possible and seal. Give the bag a good shake. It is now ready to freeze.

To Cook

1. Empty frozen ingredients into slow cooker. Add the tomatoes, coconut milk and vegetable stock if you didn't add them to the zip lock bag.
2. Cook for 5–6 hours on LOW.
3. Start making the coconut rice 30 minutes before the curry will be ready. Place the rice, coconut milk, salt and ½ cup water in a medium-sized saucepan. Bring to the boil then reduce to a simmer and cook, covered, for 15–20 minutes or until the rice has absorbed all the liquid. Remove from the heat and fluff with a fork. Serve with the curry.

Storage & Reheating

The cooked curry will keep for up to 1 week in the fridge or 2–3 months in the freezer. Cool completely before chilling or freezing. The rice will only keep for 2 days in the fridge and should not be frozen.

If cooking from frozen, defrost overnight in the fridge. Reheat the meal thoroughly in a microwave or saucepan.

White Bean Stew

Ingredients

2 cups dried white beans, soaked in cold water overnight

1 onion, chopped

1 carrot, diced

3 celery stalks, diced

3 garlic cloves, finely chopped

3 rosemary sprigs, leaves picked

3 thyme sprigs, leaves picked

1 bunch spinach, stalks removed and leaves roughly chopped

1 bunch chard or kale, stalks removed and leaves roughly chopped

2 teaspoons salt

2 x 400 g tins whole peeled tomatoes

½ teaspoon pepper

Method

Drain the beans and place in a zip lock bag along with the remaining ingredients except the salt. If you need to save freezer space or your zip lock bag isn't quite big enough, simply leave out the tinned tomatoes and add them when you start cooking. Squeeze out as much air as possible and seal. Give the bag a good shake. It is now ready to freeze.

To Cook

1. There is no need to defrost the ingredients. Simply empty the ingredients into a slow cooker along with 2.5 litres water and the tinned tomatoes if you didn't add them to the zip lock bag.
2. Cook for 6–7 hours on LOW.
3. Season with salt and serve.

Serving Suggestion

Serve with crusty bread on the side.

Storage & Reheating

The cooked stew will keep for 1 week in the fridge or 2–3 months in the freezer. Cool completely before chilling or freezing.

If cooking from frozen, defrost overnight in the fridge. Reheat the meal thoroughly in a microwave or saucepan.

'Butter' Chickpeas & Tofu

Ingredients

1 tablespoon canola, sunflower or grapeseed oil

1 onion, chopped

4 garlic cloves, finely chopped

4 cm piece ginger, finely chopped

1 bunch coriander, stalks and roots finely chopped, leaves roughly chopped, for garnish

1 tablespoon garam masala

1 tablespoon curry powder

1 teaspoon ground cardamom

1 teaspoon sweet paprika

1 teaspoon chilli powder

1 tablespoon ground coriander

400 g firm tofu, cubed, drained and wrapped in paper towel to soak up excess moisture

1 cup dried chickpeas, soaked in cold water overnight, drained

1 x 200 ml tin coconut milk

1 x 400 g tin peeled tomatoes

1 teaspoon salt

½ teaspoon pepper

1 cup raw cashews

Method

1. Heat the oil in a frying pan over medium–high heat. Sauté the onion, garlic, ginger and coriander stalks and roots for 8 minutes, stirring frequently. Add the spices and toast for a few minutes. Set the mixture aside to cool. (Alternatively, you can skip this step and just put all of the ingredients in a zip lock bag, but this really boosts the flavour.)

2. Place a zip lock bag in a bowl and add all of the ingredients except the cashews and coriander leaves to the bag. Squeeze out as much air as possible and seal the bag. Give the bag a good shake. It is now ready to store in the fridge for a couple of days before cooking. Tofu does not freeze well so we recommend you eat this meal soon.

To Cook

1. Empty the ingredients into a slow cooker.
2. Cook for 4–5 hours on LOW.
3. Stir through the cashews and cook for a further 5 minutes.
4. Garnish with the coriander leaves.

Serving Suggestion

Serve with steamed basmati rice on the side.

Storage & Reheating

The cooked curry will keep for up to 1 week in the fridge. Tofu does not freeze well so we recommend you keep this cooked dish in the fridge.

Reheat in the microwave or on the stovetop over a gentle heat in a covered saucepan.

Vegan Bolognese

Ingredients

1 onion, chopped
4 garlic cloves, chopped
3 carrots, grated
3 celery stalks, diced
10 button mushrooms, diced
1 eggplant, diced
½ butternut pumpkin, peeled, seeds removed and flesh grated
½ head cauliflower, chopped
4 oregano sprigs, leaves picked
1 bunch basil, upper stalks finely chopped, leaves picked
2 tablespoons tomato paste
2 tablespoons brown sugar
2 tablespoons olive oil
1 teaspoon salt
½ teaspoon pepper
2 x 400 g tins whole peeled tomatoes
1 cup vegetable stock

Method

1. Place the vegetables in a food processor and pulse until finely chopped.
2. Place a zip lock bag in a bowl and add all of the ingredients to the bag. If you need to save freezer space or your zip lock bag isn't quite big enough, simply leave out the tinned tomatoes and vegetable stock and add them when you start cooking. Squeeze out as much air as possible and seal. Give the bag a good shake. It is now ready to freeze.

To Cook

1. Cook from frozen. Empty the ingredients into a slow cooker. Add the tinned tomatoes if you didn't add them to the zip lock bag.
2. Cook for 7–8 hours on LOW. Season, to taste.

Serving Suggestion

Serve the vegan bolognese on top of the pasta.

Storage & Reheating

The cooked bolognese will keep for up to 1 week in the fridge or 2–3 months in the freezer. Cool completely before chilling or freezing.

If cooking from frozen, defrost overnight in fridge. Reheat thoroughly in a microwave or saucepan.

Black Beans & Rice

Ingredients

1 cup dried black beans, soaked in cold water overnight
3 garlic cloves, finely chopped
1 onion, finely chopped
1 red capsicum, finely diced
2 teaspoons ground cumin
1 teaspoon ground coriander
1 teaspoon chilli powder
½ teaspoon salt
¼ teaspoon pepper
1 x 400 g tin crushed tomatoes
1 cup long-grain rice

Method

Drain the black beans and place in a zip lock bag with the remaining ingredients except the rice. If you need to save freezer space or your zip lock bag isn't quite big enough, simply leave out the tinned tomatoes and add them when you start cooking. Squeeze out as much air as possible and seal. Give the bag a good shake. It is now ready to freeze.

To Cook

1. There is no need to defrost the ingredients. Simply empty the ingredients into a slow cooker.
2. Cook for 5–6 hours on LOW.

Storage & Reheating

This dish will keep for up to 1 week in the fridge or 2–3 months in the freezer. Cool completely before chilling or freezing.

If cooking from frozen, defrost overnight in the fridge. Reheat the meal thoroughly in a microwave or saucepan.

Sweet Potato, Pumpkin, Carrot & Split-Pea Soup

Ingredients

1 onion, chopped

1 butternut pumpkin, peeled, seeds removed and flesh cut into chunks

2 sweet potatoes, peeled and cut into large chunks

3 carrots, cut into large chunks

3 rosemary sprigs, leaves picked

½ cup split peas

1 teaspoon salt

½ teaspoon pepper

2 litres vegetable stock

Method

Place a zip lock bag in a bowl and add all of the ingredients except the vegetable stock to the bag. Squeeze out as much air as possible and seal. Give the bag a good shake. It is now ready to freeze.

To Cook

1. Empty the frozen ingredients into a slow cooker and add the vegetable stock.
2. Cook for 6 hours on LOW.
3. You can mash the soup at the end for a chunky soup or purée in a blender or food processor if you prefer a smooth soup.

Serving Suggestion

Serve with crusty bread.

Storage & Reheating

The cooked soup will keep for 1 week in the fridge or 2–3 months in the freezer. Cool completely before chilling or freezing.

If cooking from frozen, defrost overnight in the fridge. Reheat the meal thoroughly in a microwave or saucepan.

Indian Curried Eggplant

Ingredients

2 large eggplants, each chopped into 10–12 pieces and soaked in water

1 onion, chopped

3 garlic cloves, finely chopped

1 medium green chilli, finely chopped

4 cm piece ginger, finely chopped

1 bunch coriander, stalks and roots finely chopped, leaves roughly chopped

2 teaspoons ground cumin

2 teaspoons turmeric

1 teaspoon curry powder

1 teaspoon salt

½ teaspoon pepper

2 cups vegetable stock

Method

1. Place a zip lock bag in a large bowl and add the spices to the bag. Add the eggplant then seal the bag and give it a good shake to coat.
2. Add the remaining ingredients except the vegetable stock and coriander leaves. Squeeze out as much air as possible and seal. Give the bag a good shake. It is now ready to freeze.

To Cook

1. Empty the frozen ingredients into a slow cooker and add the vegetable stock.
2. Cook for 4–5 hours on LOW.
3. Garnish with the coriander leaves.

Serving Suggestion

Serve the curried eggplant with steamed rice and lemon wedges.

Storage & Reheating

This dish will keep for 1 week in the fridge or 2–3 months in the freezer. Cool completely before chilling or freezing.

To cook from frozen, defrost overnight in the fridge. Reheat thoroughly in a microwave or saucepan.

Meat-Free Week Menu

Meat-Free Week Menu

Some weeks we simply don't feel like eating any meat and sometimes our budgets need us to take a little break from it, too. This plan has family dinners that are satisfying and delicious even for the most die-hard meat eaters amongst us.

Menu

Potato Pizzas

Vegetarian Chilli

Red Lentil Dal with Greens

Pumpkin Falafel & Flatbreads

Veggie Dumplings

Pumpkin & Ricotta Cannelloni

Sesame Soba Noodles with Crisp Vegetables

Shopping List

Fruit & Veg	Dairy & Frozen	Tins, Jars & Dry Goods
6 onions	3 eggs	3 x 400 g tins whole peeled tomatoes
2 heads garlic	200 g parmesan	2 x 400 g tins crushed tomatoes
1 x 4 cm piece ginger	150 g mozzarella	2 x 400 g tins chickpeas
3 potatoes	250 g ricotta	3 x 400 g tins kidney beans
6 carrots	80 g butter	400 g red lentils
1 butternut pumpkin		
2 red capsicums		
2 corn cobs		
20 button mushrooms		
¼ white cabbage		
7 handfuls baby spinach		
1 bunch kale		
8 spring onions		
1 bunch rosemary		
2 bunches parsley		
½ bunch coriander		
1 bunch basil		
2 handfuls snow peas		
2 handfuls green beans		

Pantry Essentials		Other Ingredients
canola, sunflower or grapeseed oil	¼ tsp cayenne pepper	2 packs gyoza skins
olive oil	2 tbs chilli powder	375 g fresh pasta sheets
1.35 kg plain flour	½ tsp dried chilli flakes	500 g dried buckwheat soba noodles
4 tsp dry active yeast	1 tbs plus 3 tsp ground cumin	
2 tbs brown sugar	1½ tbs ground coriander	
1 tbs honey	1 tsp garam masala	
salt	½ tsp ground turmeric	
pepper	2 star anise	
2 tbs soy sauce	1 cinnamon stick	
1 tbs mirin	6 curry leaves	
3 tsp sesame oil	2 tbs toasted sesame seeds	
⅓ cup tahini		
2 tbs plus 1 tsp smoked paprika		

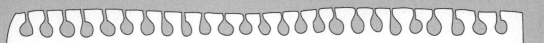

Serving Size
Each meal serves a family of 4 (approximately)

Preparation time
3½ hours

Equipment
Preparation: stand mixer (optional), sharp knives, chopping boards, kitchen scales, measuring cups and spoons, vegetable peeler, grater, mixing bowls in assorted sizes, rolling pin, whisk, mixing spoon, plastic wrap, paper towel.
Cooking: casserole dish or Dutch oven, large, heavy-based frying pan, medium and large saucepans, baking trays, ceramic or glass baking dish.
Storage: zip lock bags, airtight containers suitable for freezing, foil.

Storage & Reheating
Most of the meals in this menu are freezer friendly and can be stored for 1–3 months in the freezer.

The chilli, dal, falafel, pizza and cannelloni need to be defrosted overnight or during the day that you plan to eat them, while the dumplings can be cooked from frozen.

The sauce for the Sesame Soba Noodles with Crisp Vegetables can be made in advance and stored in a jar in the fridge for up to 2 weeks, but the veggies and noodles should be prepped just before serving, which only takes a few minutes.

All meals in this plan will last for 1 week in the fridge, except the dumplings which must be frozen until they are cooked. Once the dumplings are cooked they will last about 5 days in the fridge, but they are best cooked from frozen.

Once-A-Week Cooking Preparation

	Total	Potato Pizzas	Vegetarian Chilli	Red Lentil Dal with Greens
Pizza and Flatbread Dough				
The recipe for the Pizza Dough and the not-so-Flatbreads is the same, so make a double batch with 1.1 kg flour, 4 teaspoons dry active yeast, 4 tablespoons olive oil and 740 ml of water.				
Fresh Produce				
Onion	6		1 finely chopped	2 finely chopped
Garlic	2	4 cloves, finely chopped	6 cloves, finely chopped	3 cloves, finely chopped
Ginger	4 cm piece			
Potatoes	3	3 peeled and thinly sliced		
Carrots	6			
Pumpkin	1			
Capsicum	2		1 finely diced	
Corn	2		2 cobs, kernels stripped	
Mushrooms	20			
White cabbage	¼			
Baby spinach (handfuls)	7	reserve 3 handfuls		reserve 2 handfuls
Kale	1			1 bunch, stalks removed and leaves shredded
Spring onions (bunch)	1			
Rosemary	1	4 sprigs, leaves picked and finely chopped		
Parsley	2	1 bunch, stalks finely chopped, leaves roughly chopped		
Coriander	½			
Basil	1			
Snow peas	2			
Green beans (handfuls)	2			
Cheese				
Mozzarella	150 g			
Parmesan	200 g	100 g, grated		

Pumpkin Falafel & Flatbreads	Veggie Dumplings	Pumpkin & Ricotta Cannelloni	Sesame Soba Noodles with Crisp Vegetables
Prepare the other ingredients while the dough rises.			
1 finely chopped	2 finely chopped		
3 cloves, finely chopped	2 cloves, finely chopped		
	4 cm piece, finely chopped		
	4 grated		2 julienned
½, peeled, seeds removed and cut into chunks		½, peeled, seeds removed and cut into chunks	
			1 julienned
	20 thinly sliced		
	¼ finely shredded		
		2 handfuls, shredded	
	8 thinly sliced		
1 bunch, stalks and leaves finely chopped			
	½ bunch, finely chopped		
		1 bunch, finely chopped	
			2 handfuls, topped and tailed
			2 handfuls, topped and tailed
		150 g, grated	
		100 g, grated	

Once-A-Week Cooking Plan

1. Preheat the oven to 180°C. Place two heavy-based saucepans over medium heat.

2. Make the dough for the **Potato Pizzas** and **Pumpkin Falafel & Flatbreads**. Set aside in a warm place to rise.

3. Prepare the **Vegetarian Chilli** and **Red Lentil Dal with Greens** so they have time to cook and cool.

4. Once the pumpkin is cool, prepare the filling for the **Pumpkin & Ricotta Cannelloni** and the mixture for the **Pumpkin Falafel & Flatbreads**. Form the falafels and fry them, then fill the cannelloni and whip up the simple sauce to go over it. Bake the cannelloni.

5. Make the **Veggie Dumpling** filling so this has time to cool before filling the gyoza skins.

6. Once the dough has risen, increase the oven temperature to 200°C and divide the dough into four pieces: reserve two for the **Flatbreads** and roll the remaining two pieces into large pizza bases for the **Potato Pizzas**.

7. Top the pizzas and bake.

8. Set a frying pan over high heat and cook the **Flatbreads** for a couple of minutes each side.

9. Fill and seal the **Veggie Dumplings** before chilling and freezing or cooking.

10. Whip together the **Sesame Sauce** for the **Soba Noodles with Crisp Vegetables**. Decant and set aside in the fridge.

11. Allow all dishes to cool completely before chilling or freezing.

Potato Pizzas

Ingredients
Dough

550 g plain flour, plus extra
    for dusting

2 tablespoons olive oil

1 teaspoon salt

2 teaspoons dry active yeast

370 ml warm water

Topping

4 garlic cloves, finely chopped

4 rosemary sprigs, leaves picked
    and finely chopped

1 bunch parsley, stalks finely
    chopped, leaves roughly
    chopped

80 g butter

3 large potatoes, peeled and
    thinly sliced

3 tablespoons olive oil

1 egg, beaten

3 handfuls baby spinach

100 g parmesan, grated

Method

1. Add the flour, olive oil and salt to the bowl of a stand mixer with a dough hook attachment or large bowl. Double the quantity of all dough ingredients if you are also making the dough for the Pumpkin Falafel & Flatbreads.

2. In a jug or bowl, add the yeast to the warm water and set aside for about 10 minutes, until the mixture begins to froth. Add this to the flour and mix until a rough dough forms.

3. If you are using a stand mixer, knead the dough for 5 minutes. Alternatively, scrape the dough onto a well-floured surface and knead for about 8–10 minutes by hand until you have a smooth dough.

4. Transfer the dough to a large lightly oiled bowl, cover with plastic wrap and set aside for 2 hours or until doubled in size.

5. Add the garlic, rosemary, parsley stalks and butter to a large heavy-based frying pan over medium heat. Allow the mixture to bubble and colour slightly before adding the potato and tossing to combine. Add the olive oil and cook until the potato is nearly tender, about 8–10 minutes. Season, to taste.

6. Preheat the oven to 200°C.
7. If you have made a double quantity of dough, halve it and set aside one half, wrapped in plastic wrap, for the Pumpkin Falafel & Flatbreads. Divide the dough for the pizzas in half and roll out on a well-floured surface into large pizza bases, about 1 cm thick. Place each dough circle on a large, well-floured baking tray.
8. Brush each pizza base with a little beaten egg and scatter over the baby spinach leaves. Spread the potato mixture on top and sprinkle over the parsley. Top with the parmesan and season.
9. Bake for 15–20 minutes or until the cheese is golden and the edges are crisp and golden brown.

Serving Suggestion
Serve with a fresh green salad.

Storage & Reheating
Allow to cool completely before chilling or freezing. The pizzas will keep for 1 week in the fridge or 1 month in the freezer.

To cook from frozen, remove from the freezer 10 minutes before baking, then follow step 9 to cook.

Vegetarian Chilli

Ingredients

3 tablespoons oil
1 onion, finely chopped
6 garlic cloves, finely chopped
1 red capsicum, finely diced
1 tablespoon ground cumin
2 tablespoons chilli powder
1 tablespoon ground coriander

2 tablespoons smoked paprika
¼ teaspoon cayenne pepper
2 x 400 g tins crushed tomatoes
2 tablespoons brown sugar
3 x 400 g tins kidney beans
2 corn cobs, kernels stripped

Method

1. Heat the oil in a heavy-based casserole dish or Dutch oven over medium heat. Add the onion, garlic and capsicum and cook until softened, about 5 minutes. Push the vegetables to one side of the dish then add the spices to the other side. Toast the spices for about one minute before stirring through the vegetables.
2. Add 2 cups water then bring the mixture to the boil and allow to cook for 5 minutes. Add the tomato and sugar and simmer for 20 minutes. Add the kidney beans and corn kernels and cook for 5 minutes. Season the chilli, to taste.

Serving Suggestion

Serve on top of a bowl of tortilla chips or steamed rice with coriander leaves, lime juice, grated mozzarella and sour cream.

Storage & Reheating

Allow to cool completely before chilling or freezing. The chilli will keep for 1 week in the fridge or 3 months in the freezer.

To cook from frozen, defrost overnight in the fridge. Reheat thoroughly in a microwave or saucepan.

Red Lentil Dal with Greens

Ingredients

400 g red lentils, rinsed
2 tablespoons oil
2 onions, finely chopped
3 garlic cloves, finely chopped
½ teaspoon ground turmeric
1 teaspoon ground coriander
1 teaspoon garam masala
1 teaspoon ground cumin

½ teaspoon dried chilli flakes
2 star anise
1 large cinnamon stick
6 curry leaves
1 x 400 g tin whole peeled
    tomatoes
1 bunch kale, stalks removed and
    leaves shredded
2 handfuls baby spinach

Method

1. Place the lentils and 1 litre water in a large saucepan. Bring to the boil then reduce to a simmer and cook for 15 minutes until the lentils are soft. Drain and set aside.
2. Heat the oil in a large saucepan over medium heat. Add the onion and garlic and sauté until the onion is translucent and lightly coloured. Add the spices and curry leaves and cook for 2 minutes until fragrant. Add the tomatoes, stir to combine and cook for 10 minutes. Stir in the red lentils, shredded kale and spinach.
3. Simmer and cook for 15 minutes. If the mixture becomes a little dry, add a couple of tablespoons of water. Season, to taste.

Serving Suggestion

Serve with a side of basmati or brown rice.

Storage & Reheating

Allow to cool completely before chilling or freezing. The dal will keep for 1 week in the fridge or 3 months in the freezer.

To cook from frozen, defrost overnight in the fridge. Reheat thoroughly in a microwave or saucepan.

Pumpkin Falafel & Flatbreads

Ingredients

Flatbreads

550 g plain flour

2 tablespoons olive oil

1 teaspoon salt

2 teaspoons dry active yeast

370 ml warm water

Falafel

½ butternut pumpkin, peeled, seeds removed and cut into large chunks

80 ml canola, sunflower or grapeseed oil

2 x 400 g tins chickpeas

1 onion, finely chopped

3 garlic cloves, finely chopped

1 bunch parsley, stalks and leaves finely chopped

2 teaspoons ground cumin

1 teaspoon ground coriander

1 teaspoon smoked paprika

1 egg, lightly beaten

1 teaspoon salt

½ teaspoon pepper

250 g plain flour (you may not need the full amount)

Method

1. To make the dough, add the flour, olive oil and salt to the bowl of a stand mixer with a dough hook attachment or large bowl. Double the quantity of all dough ingredients if you are also making the dough for the Potato Pizzas.

2. In a jug or bowl, add the yeast to the warm water and set aside for about 10 minutes, until the mixture begins to froth. Add this to the flour and mix until a rough dough forms.

3. If you are using a stand mixer knead the dough for 5 minutes. Alternatively, scrape the dough onto a well-floured surface and knead for about 8–10 minutes by hand until you have a smooth dough.

4. Transfer the dough to a large lightly oiled bowl, cover with plastic wrap and set aside for 2 hours or until doubled in size.

5. Preheat the oven to 180°C.

6. To make the falafel, drizzle the pumpkin with 1 tablespoon oil and roast in the oven until tender, about 45 minutes. Set aside to cool.
7. Whizz all of the falafel ingredients except the flour in a food processor. Once the mixture is smooth, start adding the flour little by little until you have a soft, pliable dough-like consistency. Set aside.
8. Flatbreads: Scrape the risen dough onto a floured surface and wrap half in plastic wrap (if reserving for the Potato Pizzas). Divide the remaining dough into 16 pieces and roll each into a flat round, about ½ cm thick.
9. Heat a little oil in a griddle pan or frying pan over medium heat. Add 1 dough circle and cook for 2–3 minutes on each side. Set aside and repeat with the remaining dough rounds.
10. To cook the falafel, place a heavy-based frying pan over medium–high heat and add the remaining oil. Using wet hands, roll golf ball-sized balls of falafel mix. Flatten slightly, pop in the hot oil and fry until golden brown on each side, about 2–3 minutes.

Serving Suggestion

Line a flatbread with a little Greek yoghurt, a couple of cucumber slices, diced tomatoes, falafels with fresh mint scattered on top then fold the flatbread over everything.

Storage & Reheating

Allow the falafel to cool completely before chilling or freezing. They will keep for 1 week in the fridge or 3 months in the freezer. The flatbreads will keep in an airtight container for 5 days in the pantry, 1 week in the fridge or 2 months in the freezer.

If cooking from frozen, defrost the falafel overnight in the fridge. Reheat thoroughly in a 180°C oven. Defrost the flatbreads and reheat in lightly oiled frying pan over medium heat.

Veggie Dumplings

Ingredients

1 cup canola, sunflower or grapeseed oil

20 button mushrooms, thinly sliced

4 cm piece ginger, finely chopped

2 garlic cloves, finely chopped

2 onions, finely chopped

¼ white cabbage, finely shredded

4 carrots, grated

8 spring onions, thinly sliced

1½ teaspoons salt

1 teaspoon white pepper

2 teaspoons sesame oil

½ bunch coriander, stalks and leaves finely chopped

2 packs gyoza skins

Method

1. Heat 1 teaspoon of the oil in a large frying pan or wok over medium heat. Add the mushrooms, ginger, garlic and onion and sauté until the onion is soft and translucent. Add the cabbage, carrot and spring onion and cook for about 6–8 minutes, stirring frequently, until the vegetables have softened. Season with the salt and white pepper, to taste.

2. Transfer the mixture to a colander and drain any excess liquid. Place the mixture in a large bowl and add the sesame oil and coriander. Stir to combine.

3. Lay out the gyoza skins and place a small bowl of water on the kitchen bench. Place 1 tablespoon of the mixture on one side of each gyoza skin, leaving a clean edge. Dip your finger in the water and run along the edge of the gyoza skin before folding the other side over the filling and sealing the dumpling. Crimp the tops. This should yield approximately 60+ dumplings.

*   **At this point the dumplings can be frozen in zip lock bags until you are ready to cook them. Dumplings should be cooked from frozen and not defrosted.**

4. Heat a large non-stick frying pan with a fitted lid over medium heat. Add the remaining oil to generously coat the bottom of the pan. When the oil is hot, place the dumplings in the bottom of the

pan. You may need to cook the dumplings in batches. Allow the bottoms of the dumplings to brown, about 3–4 minutes.

5. Add ½ cup water to the pan (or ¼ cup if you are cooking the dumplings in batches) and pop the lid on. Keep the lid on until the water has steamed up and evaporated. The steam will cook the tops of the dumplings. Remove the lid and allow the dumplings to cook for a further 2–3 minutes.

Serving Suggestion

Serve with steamed rice and a little soy sauce for dipping the dumplings.

Storage & Reheating

Freeze after step 3 or, if cooked, allow to cool completely before chilling. The cooked dumplings will keep for 1 week in the fridge. Do not freeze cooked dumplings.

To cook from frozen, you can boil, steam or pan-fry the dumplings.

Pumpkin & Ricotta Cannelloni

Ingredients

½ butternut pumpkin, peeled, seeds removed and cut into chunks

1 tablespoon oil

2 x 400 g tins whole peeled tomatoes

1 bunch basil, leaves finely chopped

250 g ricotta

150 g mozzarella (plus extra for sprinkling)

1 egg, lightly beaten

2 handfuls baby spinach, shredded

375 g fresh pasta sheets

100 g parmesan, grated

Method

1. Preheat the oven to 180°C. Lightly grease a ceramic baking dish.
2. Drizzle the pumpkin with the oil and roast in the dish until tender, about 45 minutes. Transfer to a bowl and mash. Set aside to cool.
3. To make the sauce, place a medium-sized saucepan over high heat and add the tinned tomatoes and half the basil leaves. Season, to taste. Bring to the boil then reduce to a simmer and cook until reduced by one-third, about 10–15 minutes. Remove from the heat.
4. In a large bowl, mix the ricotta, mozzarella, egg, spinach and mashed pumpkin. Season with salt and pepper, to taste.
5. Lay out the pasta sheets and place 2 tablespoons of the pumpkin mixture at the base of each sheet and roll up into a tube. Lay each cannelloni in the baking dish. Top with the prepared sauce and grated parmesan.
6. Bake for 30 minutes, then cover with foil and bake for a further 15 minutes.

Serving Suggestion

Serve with a fresh green salad.

Storage & Reheating

Allow to cool completely before chilling or freezing. The cannelloni will keep for 1 week in the fridge or 2 months in the freezer.

If cooking from frozen, defrost overnight in the fridge. Cover with foil and bake in a 180°C oven for 30 minutes until thoroughly reheated.

Sesame Soba Noodles with Crisp Vegetables

Ingredients
Sauce

⅓ cup of tahini

1 teaspoon sesame oil

1 tablespoon honey, agave or other liquid sweetener

2 tablespoons soy sauce

1 tablespoon mirin or rice vinegar

1 cm piece ginger, grated (optional)

2 tablespoons toasted sesame seeds, for garnish (optional)

500 g dried buckwheat soba noodles

2 carrots, julienned

1 red capsicum, julienned

2 handfuls snow peas, topped and tailed

2 handfuls green beans, topped and tailed

Method

1. To make the sauce whisk all of the ingredients in a small bowl. Adjust the flavours, to taste. The sauce should be a pourable consistency.
2. Bring a large saucepan of water to a rolling boil. Add the soba noodles and stir to make sure all the noodles are submerged and not sticking together. Cook for about 2 minutes until tender. Remove the noodles from the water and add the prepared veggies to refresh them. Drain.
3. Refresh the noodles under cold running water until they are cool enough to handle. Divide the noodles and vegetables among bowls and top with the prepared sauce.

Storage & Reheating

This isn't a freezer meal but you can make the sauce ahead of time and store in a jar in the fridge for up to 2 weeks.

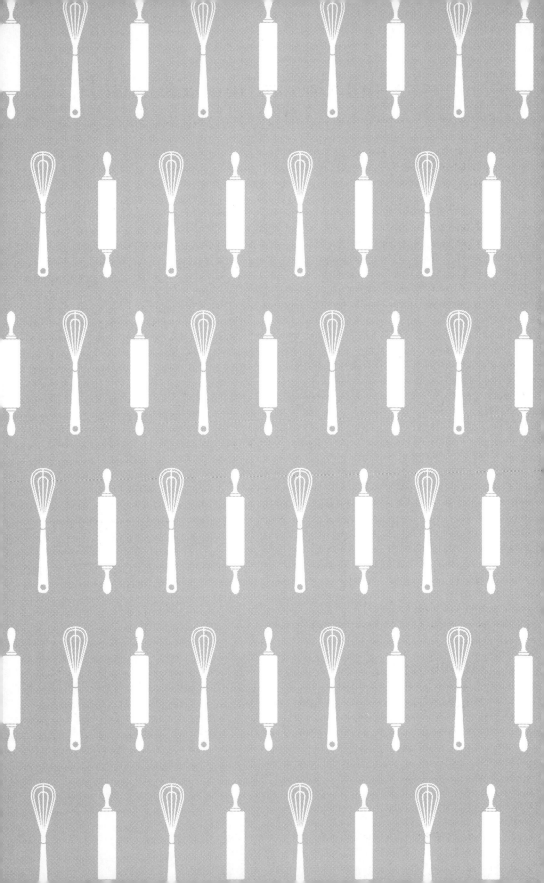

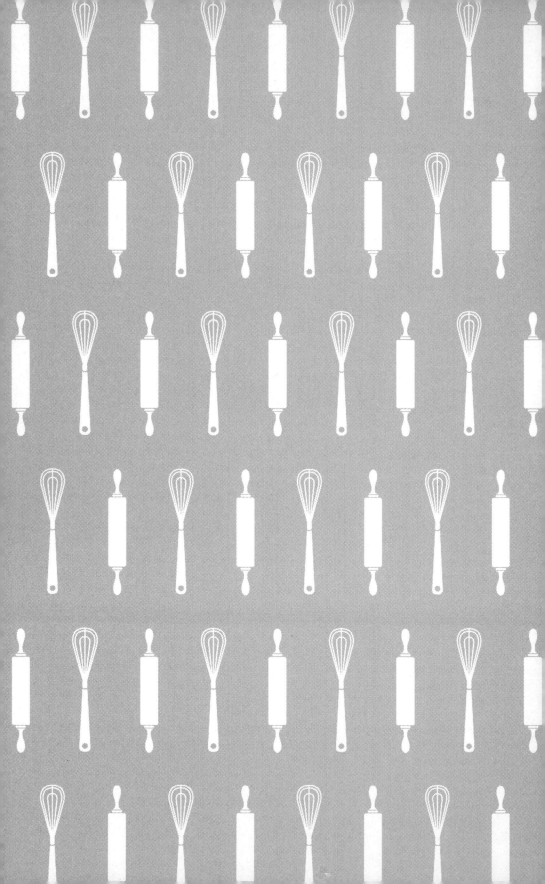

One Month of Wholesome School Lunches

One Month of Wholesome School Lunches

This plan prepares one month of school lunches for two children with reasonable appetites. Increase the quantity of each recipe by half for each additional child. With five different menu items, this means eight serves per recipe covering 20 school days over four weeks. Everything is freezer-friendly and you can easily have a different lunch every day just by cooking each lunch from frozen alongside whatever else you might be cooking in your oven the night before.

MamaBaker Hannah says:

> "I made a promise to myself that this was the year I was going to get organised to take the stress out of school lunchbox preparation. I found the process of preparing the recipes very straightforward and, although it took me a little longer (note to self, do the plan while the kids are at school!) than the suggested time frame, I was thrilled with the results. I've been dipping into the freezer stash for after-school snacks, with the veggie-packed sausage rolls being a winner for my girls."

Menu

Cheesy Chicken Buns

Herby Ham & Olive Focaccia

Bacon & Zucchini Slice

Veggie-Packed Sausage Rolls

Herbed Chicken Fingers

Shopping List

Meat & Fish	Fruit & Veg	Dairy & Frozen
2.4 kg chicken breasts 800 g pork mince 6 rashers bacon 5 slices ham	1 onion 3 carrots 1 head broccoli 4 zucchinis 2 bunches English spinach 1 bunch parsley 3 thyme sprigs 3 rosemary sprigs 1 bunch basil 1 apple	300 g tasty cheese 160 g parmesan 9 eggs 1 tbs butter 1 cup milk 6 frozen puff pastry sheets
Tins, Jars & Dry Goods	**Pantry Essentials**	**Other Ingredients**
100 g pitted Kalamata olives 2 cups breadcrumbs	canola, sunflower or grapeseed oil olive oil 1.5 kg plain flour 4½ tsp dry active yeast 2 tsp baking powder 1 tsp sugar salt pepper 3 tbs Worcestershire sauce 2 tbs tomato sauce (ketchup) 1 tbs dried oregano	none

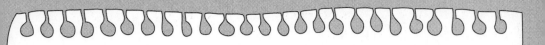

Serving Size
Each recipe makes approximately 8 serves

Preparation time
3 hours

Equipment
Preparation: stand or hand-held mixer, sharp knives, chopping boards suitable for vegetables and meat, kitchen scales, measuring cups and spoons, vegetable peeler, grater, mixing bowls in assorted sizes, rolling pin, whisk, mixing spoon.
Cooking: baking tray, 25 cm x 15 cm slice tin.
Storage: zip lock bags or airtight containers suitable for freezing.

Storage & Reheating
All of these recipes are freezer friendly. A few of the items can be prepared and baked individually as needed.

The Cheesy Chicken Buns, Herbed Chicken Fingers and Veggie-Packed Sausage Rolls can be prepared ahead of time but, to stay fresh-tasting, they should be frozen or chilled prior to baking. Individual portions can then be cooked the night before they are needed.

The Bacon & Zucchini Slice and Herby Ham & Olive Focaccia are easy to prepare and can be cut into portions before being frozen. When needed, defrost and re-bake to improve the texture. These cooked items will keep for one week in the fridge or one month in the freezer.

Once-A-Week Cooking Preparation

	Total	Cheesy Chicken Buns	Herby Ham & Olive Focaccia	Bacon & Zucchini Slice
Fresh Produce				
Onion	1			
Carrots	3			
Broccoli	1			
Zucchini	4			4 grated
English spinach (bunches)	2	1 bunch, stalks removed, leaves finely chopped		
Parsley	1	½ bunch, leaves and stalks finely chopped		
Thyme (sprigs)	3		3 sprigs, leaves picked and finely chopped	
Rosemary (sprigs)	3		3 sprigs, leaves picked and finely chopped	
Basil	1		½ bunch, leaves picked and finely chopped	
Apple	1			
Cheese				
Tasty cheese	300 g	200 g, grated		100 g, grated
Parmesan	160 g		80 g, grated	
Meat				
Chicken breasts	2.4 kg	600 g cut into bite-sized pieces		
Bacon	6			6 rashers, thinly sliced
Ham	5		5 slices, shredded	

Veggie-Packed Sausage Rolls	Herbed Chicken Fingers
1 finely chopped	
3 grated	
1 head cut into florets, stalk peeled and grated	
1 bunch, stalks removed, leaves finely chopped	
	½ bunch, finely chopped
	½ bunch, finely chopped
1 grated	
80 g, grated	
	1.8 kg – each breast cut into 8 long strips

Once-A-Week Cooking Plan

1. Prepare the doughs for the **Cheesy Chicken Buns** and the **Herby Ham & Olive Focaccia** and set aside to rise.

2. Defrost the puff pastry for the **Veggie-Packed Sausage Rolls**

3. Prepare the filling for the **Cheesy Chicken Buns** and set aside to cool.

4. Preheat the oven to 180°C and make the **Bacon & Zucchini Slice**. Bake for 30–40 minutes.

5. Prepare the vegetables for the **Veggie-Packed Sausage Rolls** and allow to cool before combining with the meat mixture.

6. Set up a production line of flour, egg and breadcrumbs and prepare the **Herbed Chicken Fingers**.

7. Once the dough is ready, make the **Herby Ham & Olive Focaccia** and bake.

8. Roll out the dough for the **Cheesy Chicken Buns**, fill, seal and bake.

9. Fill the puff pastry with the **Veggie Packed Sausage Rolls** mixture, seal, cut, glaze and bake.

10. Allow all items to cool completely before placing in the fridge or freezer for storage.

Cheesy Chicken Buns

Dough

700 g plain flour, plus extra for
  dusting
1½ teaspoons salt

2½ teaspoons dry active yeast
400 ml warm water

Filling

1 tablespoon canola, sunflower or
  grapeseed oil
600 g chicken breasts, cut into
  bite-sized pieces
1 bunch English spinach, stalks
  removed, leaves finely chopped
1 tablespoon butter

1 tablespoon flour
1 cup milk
200 g tasty cheese, grated
½ bunch parsley, leaves and stalks
  finely chopped
1 teaspoon salt
½ teaspoon pepper

Method

1. To make the dough, place the flour and salt in the bowl of a stand
   mixer or large bowl.
2. In a separate jug or bowl, add the yeast to the warm water and set
   aside for 10 minutes until the mixture begins to froth. Pour into the
   flour and mix until a rough dough forms.
3. If you are using a stand mixer, knead the dough for 5 minutes.
   Alternatively, if you are making the dough by hand, scrape
   the dough onto a well-floured surface and knead for about
   8–10 minutes.
4. Transfer the dough to a large lightly oiled bowl, cover with plastic
   wrap and set aside for 2 hours or until doubled in size.
5. To make the filling, heat the oil in a medium-sized saucepan
   over medium–high heat. Add the chicken and cook, stirring,
   until browned, then add the spinach leaves and cook until wilted.
   Transfer the mixture to a bowl and set aside in the fridge to cool.
6. To make the béchamel sauce, rinse out the saucepan and return to
   medium heat. Add the butter and allow it to melt and froth. Add the
   flour and stir constantly until the mixture resembles wet sand. Add

the milk and whisk to combine. Whisk constantly as the mixture begins to bubble. Simmer for 3–4 minutes or until the sauce thickens. Season to taste and set aside to cool for a few minutes.

7. Add the béchamel sauce and grated cheese to the chicken mixture. Stir to combine.
8. Preheat the oven to 180°C.
9. Punch down the dough and divide into 16 pieces. Roll each piece into a ball and then flatten with a rolling pin to about 1 cm thick.
10. Place a dessert spoon of the chicken mixture in the centre of each dough round. Pull the edges of the dough around the filling and squeeze together to seal.

★   **At this point, the buns can be frozen. They will keep for up to 2 months unbaked in the freezer.**

11. Place each bun seam side up on a baking tray lined with baking paper. Although it makes sense to place them seam side down, the chances of the buns busting a leak are pretty good, so they look much better leaking volcanically from the top rather than oozing all over the bottom.
12. Bake for 15–20 minutes or until golden brown.

Storage & Reheating

Allow to cool completely before chilling or freezing. The cooked buns will keep for up to 1 week in the fridge or 1 month in the freezer.

For best results, freeze rolls unbaked. Bake from frozen. Simply cook individual portions the night before they're needed.

Herby Ham & Olive Focaccia

Ingredients

550 g plain flour

1 teaspoon salt

80 ml olive oil, plus extra for greasing

3 thyme sprigs, leaves picked and finely chopped

3 rosemary sprigs, leaves picked and finely chopped

½ bunch basil, leaves picked and finely chopped

1 tablespoon dried oregano

½ teaspoon pepper

2 teaspoons dry active yeast

1 teaspoon sugar

370 ml warm water

5 slices ham, shredded

100 g pitted Kalamata olives, halved

80 g parmesan, grated

Method

1. To make the dough, place the flour, salt, 3 tablespoons of the olive oil, fresh herbs, dried oregano and pepper in the bowl of a stand mixer or large bowl.

2. In a separate jug or bowl, add the yeast to the warm water and set aside for 10 minutes until the mixture begins to froth. Pour into the flour and mix until a rough dough forms.

3. If you are using a stand mixer, knead the dough for 5 minutes. Alternatively, if you are making the dough by hand, scrape the dough onto a well-floured surface and knead for about 8–10 minutes.

4. Transfer the dough to a large lightly oiled bowl, cover with plastic wrap and set aside for 1–1½ hours or until doubled in size.

5. Preheat the oven to 200°C. Generously grease a baking tray with olive oil.

6. Place the dough on the baking tray and using your hands, punch and spread the dough until it forms a rectangle about 2 cm thick. Poke holes in the dough about 2 cm apart. Place pieces of ham or olives alternately in the holes. Brush the focaccia with the remaining olive oil and sprinkle with parmesan.

7. Bake for 15–18 minutes or until puffed and golden brown. Cut into 8 portions.

Storage & Reheating

Allow to cool completely before chilling or freezing. The cooked focaccia will keep for up to 1 week in the fridge or 1 month in the freezer.

To cook from frozen, simply re-bake in a warm oven to improve the texture.

Bacon & Zucchini Slice

Ingredients

6 rashers bacon, thinly sliced

4 zucchinis, grated

5 eggs, beaten

100 g tasty cheese, grated

1 tablespoon olive oil, plus extra
for greasing

150 g plain flour

2 teaspoons baking powder

1 teaspoon salt

½ teaspoon pepper

Method

1. Preheat the oven to 180°C. Lightly oil and line a 25 cm x 15 cm slice tin with baking paper.
2. Fry the bacon in a frying pan over medium heat for a few minutes. Drain the excess oil and transfer the bacon to a large bowl.
3. Return the pan to the heat and gently cook the zucchini for 5 minutes, stirring frequently. Add it to the bowl with the bacon and set aside to cool.
4. Add the beaten egg, grated cheese and olive oil to the mixture and stir to combine. Fold in the flour and season with the salt and pepper.
5. Pour the mixture into the prepared tin and bake for 30–40 minutes or until golden brown on top.

Storage & Reheating

Allow to cool completely before cutting into 8 large portions or 16 small portions. The slice will keep for up to 1 week in the fridge or 1 month in the freezer.

To cook from frozen, defrost overnight in the fridge, then warm through in an oven preheated to 180°C to improve the texture.

Veggie-Packed Sausage Rolls

Ingredients

1 tablespoon canola, sunflower or grapeseed oil

1 onion, finely chopped

1 head broccoli, cut into florets, stalk peeled and grated

800 g pork mince

3 carrots, grated

1 bunch English spinach, stalks removed, leaves finely chopped

1 apple, grated

2 eggs

80 g parmesan, grated

3 tablespoons Worcestershire sauce

2 tablespoons tomato sauce (ketchup)

½ teaspoon salt

½ teaspoon pepper

6 puff pastry sheets, defrosted

Method

1. Heat the oil in a large saucepan over medium heat. Add the onion and sauté until translucent. Add the broccoli florets and grated stalk and allow to cook for a few minutes. Turn the heat up to high, add 3 tablespoons of water and place the lid on (this steams the broccoli). Allow to steam for 2 minutes. Remove the lid. Remove from the heat and set aside to cool.

2. In a large bowl, combine the pork, carrot, spinach, apple, 1 egg, grated parmesan, Worcestershire sauce, tomato sauce and seasoning. Add the onion and broccoli mixture and mix with your hands to combine.

3. Cut the pastry squares in half to form long rectangles. Divide the mixture between the 12 rectangles. Form the meat mixture into long, even sausages down the centre of each pastry sheet. Take one edge and roll it tightly over the meat, rolling until the meat is totally encased in pastry. Repeat with the remaining pastry and mixture. Cut each sausage roll in half.

*   **At this point, you can freeze the uncooked sausage rolls.**

4. Preheat the oven to 180°C.

5. Lightly beat the remaining egg. Place the sausage rolls at least 3 cm apart on a baking tray lined with baking paper. Brush the tops of the sausage rolls with the beaten egg.
6. Bake for about 20 minutes or until puffed up and golden brown.

Storage & Reheating

For best results, chill or freeze the sausage rolls uncooked. They will keep for up to 1 week in the fridge or 2 months in the freezer. If cooked, allow to cool completely before chilling or freezing. Cooked sausage rolls will keep for up to 1 week in the fridge or 1 month in the freezer. Bake uncooked/cooked sausage rolls from frozen. Pop individual portions in the oven to bake the night before they're needed.

Herbed Chicken Fingers

Ingredients

75 g plain flour

1.8 kg chicken breasts, each cut into 8 long strips

½ bunch parsley, leaves finely chopped

½ bunch basil, leaves finely chopped

2 cups breadcrumbs

1 teaspoon salt

½ teaspoon pepper

2 eggs, beaten

½ cup canola, sunflower or grapeseed oil

Method

1. In a large bowl, combine the flour and chicken and toss with your hands to coat. In another bowl, combine the herbs with the breadcrumbs, salt and pepper.

2. Dip the chicken in the beaten egg and then into the breadcrumb mixture. Toss and press lightly on each side to adhere the crumbs.

★ **At this point, the chicken fingers can be chilled or frozen and cooked as needed.**

3. Heat the oil in a medium-sized heavy-based frying pan over medium–high heat. Cook the chicken, in batches of no more than 5–6 pieces at a time, for 2 minutes on each side or until golden. Drain on paper towel and set aside to cool.

Storage & Reheating

The uncooked chicken fingers will keep for up to 3 days in the fridge or 2 months in the freezer. If cooked, allow to cool completely before chilling or freezing. The fingers can be stored in the fridge for up to 1 week or up to 2 months in the freezer. For best results, freeze uncooked. Defrost in the fridge overnight then simply cook in batches.

High Protein,
Low Carb

High Protein, Low Carb

This menu is for families keen to have a week of lighter carb intake. The plan isn't according to any particular school of thought and, we hope, will be appealing to everyone. Even if low carb isn't an issue for you, this menu makes a lovely week's worth of dinners for the warmer summer months when a soup or heavy stew just won't do.

Menu

Turkey Meatloaf

Tuna Quinoa Bake

Loaded Frittata

Baked Caprese Chicken

Marinated Salmon with Quinoa

Japanese-Style Steak Salad

Indian-Spiced Chicken & Cauliflower 'Rice'

Shopping List

Meat & Fish

700 g turkey mince
800 g salmon fillet
1 kg chicken breasts
    (or x4)
6 slices lean ham
700 g eye fillet steak

Fruit & Veg

2 onions
2 heads garlic
8 cm piece ginger
3 carrots
1 bunch celery
1 zucchini
2 heads broccoli
3 handfuls green beans
¼ red cabbage
1 head cauliflower
½ bunch kale
8 handfuls baby spinach
12 button mushrooms
1 punnet cherry
    tomatoes
2 cucumbers
1 bunch spring onions
1 cup beansprouts
1 bunch basil
1 bunch parsley
1 lemon

Dairy & Frozen

1 cup milk
7 egg whites
3 whole eggs
250 g cottage cheese
100 g Swiss cheese
350 g mozzarella
1 cup frozen peas

Tins, Jars & Dry Goods

400 g tin tuna in spring
    water
¾ cup rolled oats
1½ cups quinoa

Pantry Essentials

canola, sunflower or
    grapeseed oil
olive oil
700 ml vegetable
stock
2 tbs rice flour
½ tsp brown sugar
salt
pepper
1 cup tomato sauce
    (ketchup)
1 tbs chilli sauce
4 tbs plus 1 tsp low-
    sodium soy sauce

3 tbs plus 1 teaspoon
    mirin
2 tbs rice vinegar
1 tbs toasted sesame seeds
2 tsp sweet paprika
pinch of cayenne pepper
2 tsp ground cumin
1 tsp ground coriander
1 tsp garam masala
½ tsp turmeric
½ tsp freshly ground
    nutmeg

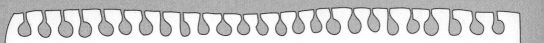

Serving Size
Each meal serves a family of 4 (approximately)

Preparation time
2.5 hours

Equipment
Preparation: food processor, sharp knives, chopping boards suitable for vegetables and fruit, meat and fish, kitchen scales, measuring cups and spoons, vegetable peeler, grater, citrus juicer, mixing bowls in assorted sizes, whisk, mixing spoon.

Cooking: large, heavy-based frying pan, medium-sized and large saucepans, 2 baking dishes, 2 pie dishes.

Storage: zip lock bags, airtight containers suitable for freezing, foil.

Storage & Reheating
For this plan, please refer to individual recipes for storage instructions for chilling and freezing as each meal is quite different.

Once-A-Week Cooking Preparation

	Total	Turkey Meatloaf	Tuna Quinoa Bake	Loaded Frittata
Fresh Produce				
Onion	2	1 finely chopped	1 finely chopped	
Garlic	2	4 cloves, finely chopped	2 cloves, finely chopped	
Ginger	8 cm piece			
Carrots	3	3 grated		
Celery	1	2 stalks, finely diced	4 stalks, finely diced	
Zucchini	1	1 grated		
Broccoli	2			1 head, florets finely chopped, stalk peeled and finely diced
Green beans (handfuls)	3		2 handfuls, topped and tailed	
Red cabbage	¼			
Cauliflower	1			
Kale	½			
Baby spinach leaves (handfuls)	8			2 handfuls
Button mushrooms	12	12 thinly sliced		
Cucumbers	2			
Spring onions (bunch)	1	6 thinly sliced		
Basil	1			
Parsley	1	½ bunch, finely chopped		
Lemon	½			
Cheese				
Swiss cheese	100 g			100 g, grated
Mozzarella	350 g		100 g, grated	
Meat & Fish				
Salmon	800 g			
Chicken breasts	1 kg			
Lean ham	6			6 slices, diced

Baked Caprese Chicken	Marinated Salmon with Quinoa	Japanese-Style Steak Salad	Indian-Spiced Chicken & Cauliflower 'Rice'
3 cloves, finely chopped	1 clove, grated		3 cloves, finely chopped
	4 cm piece, grated	4 cm piece, grated	
		1 head, florets chopped, stalk peeled and thinly sliced	
		1 handful, topped and tailed	
		¼ finely shredded	
			1 head, florets chopped
	½ bunch, stalks removed and leaves finely shredded		
4 handfuls, shredded		2 handfuls	
		2 cut into long batons	
1 bunch, leaves picked			
	½ juiced		
250 g, thinly sliced			
	800 g fillet, cut into into 4 pieces		
500 g (2 breasts) butterflied into 4 pieces			500 g (2 breasts) butterflied into 4 pieces

Once-A-Week Cooking Plan

1. Preheat the oven to 180°C.

2. Combine the ingredients for the **Turkey Meatloaf** and bake.

3. Prepare the **Tuna Quinoa Bake** and **Loaded Frittata**. Bake alongside the **Meatloaf**.

4. Prepare the **Baked Caprese Chicken** and bake alongside the other dishes.

5. If cooking the salmon for the **Marinated Salmon with Quinoa**, do this now. Otherwise freeze it and the quinoa separately, and defrost and cook on the day of consumption.

6. Also, you can decide whether to cook the steak for the **Japanese-Style Steak Salad** now and chill or freeze. Otherwise, it can be frozen uncooked and defrosted then cooked quickly on the day of consumption.

7. Prepare the spice mixture for the **Indian-Spiced Chicken & Cauliflower 'Rice'** and rub into the meat. If choosing to cook and then chill, do this now. Otherwise, place the uncooked marinated chicken in a zip lock bag and freeze.

8. Prepare the cauliflower rice for the **Indian-Spiced Chicken & Cauliflower 'Rice'** and set aside in the fridge until needed.

9. Allow all cooked dishes to cool completely before chilling or freezing.

Turkey Meatloaf

Ingredients

1 tablespoon olive oil, plus extra for greasing

4 garlic cloves, finely chopped

1 onion, finely chopped

3 carrots, grated

2 celery stalks, finely diced

1 zucchini, grated

12 button mushrooms, thinly sliced

700 g turkey mince

¾ cup rolled oats (substitute almond meal for higher protein)

½ bunch parsley, finely chopped

6 spring onions, thinly sliced

2 egg whites

1 cup tomato sauce (ketchup)

1 tablespoon chilli sauce

1 teaspoon sweet paprika

1 teaspoon ground cumin

1 teaspoon salt

½ teaspoon black pepper

Method

1. Preheat the oven to 180°C. Line a loaf tin with greased foil.
2. Heat the oil in a large saucepan over medium heat. Sauté the onion and garlic until softened, then add the carrot and celery and cook, stirring frequently, for 5 minutes. Add the zucchini and mushrooms and cook for a further 5 minutes. Set aside to cool.
3. Combine the remaining ingredients in a large bowl. Add the cooked vegetables and mix well.
4. Press the mixture into the prepared loaf tin and smooth the top with your hands. Spread the remaining tomato sauce over the top.

★ **At this point, the uncooked meatloaf can be frozen.**

5. Bake for 1–1 hour 15 minutes or until the top is caramelised and the centre is cooked through. Allow to stand for 15–20 minutes to firm up before slicing and serving.

Serving Suggestion

Serve with lightly steamed buttered vegetables.

Storage & Reheating

The uncooked meatloaf will keep for 3–4 days in the fridge or up to 2 months in the freezer. Once cooked, allow to cool completely before chilling or freezing. The meatloaf will keep for 1 week in the fridge or 2 months in the freezer.

Defrost overnight in the fridge. Follow step 5 to cook the meatloaf or reheat in a 170°C oven for 30–40 minutes.

Tuna Quinoa Bake

Ingredients

700 ml vegetable stock

¾ cup quinoa

1 tablespoon olive oil, plus extra for greasing

1 onion, finely chopped

4 celery stalks, finely diced

2 garlic cloves, finely chopped

2 tablespoons rice flour or other equivalent gluten-free flour

1 cup milk

2 handfuls green beans, topped and tailed

400 g tinned tuna in spring water, drained

100 g mozzarella, grated

½ teaspoon freshly ground nutmeg

1 teaspoon sweet paprika

Method

1. Preheat the oven to 180°C. Lightly grease a ceramic or glass baking dish.
2. Place the stock and quinoa in a medium-sized saucepan and bring to a simmer over medium–high heat. Reduce the heat and cook, covered, for 15 minutes.
3. Heat the oil in a heavy-based saucepan over medium heat and sauté the onion, celery and garlic for 10 minutes. Add the flour and paprika, cook, stirring frequently, for 3 minutes. Add the milk and nutmeg to the pan and stir to combine. Simmer for 5–7 minutes until the sauce has thickened. Add the cooked quinoa and tuna and stir to combine. Season, to taste.
4. Pour the mixture into the prepared baking dish and sprinkle over the cheese.
5. Bake for 20–30 minutes until the top is bubbling and golden.

Serving Suggestion

Serve with a crisp green salad.

Storage & Reheating

Allow to cool completely before chilling or freezing. The cooked bake will keep for up to 1 week in the fridge or 2 months in the freezer.

Reheat from frozen in a preheated 180°C oven until heated through.

Loaded Frittata

Ingredients

oil, for greasing

5 egg whites

3 whole eggs

100 g Swiss cheese, grated

1 head broccoli, florets finely chopped, stalk peeled and finely diced

6 slices lean ham, diced

250 g cottage cheese

1 cup frozen peas

2 handfuls baby spinach

¼ teaspoon salt

¼ teaspoon pepper

Method

1. Preheat the oven to 180°C. Grease a 20 cm x 30 cm ceramic or glass baking dish with a little oil.
2. Whisk the egg whites and whole eggs in a large bowl. Add the remaining ingredients and stir well to combine. Pour the mixture into the prepared dish
3. Bake for 45 minutes or until set. Allow to cool for 10 minutes before serving.

Serving Suggestion

Serve with bite-sized roasted sweet potatoes.

Storage & Reheating

Allow to cool completely before chilling or freezing. The frittata will keep, well wrapped, for up to 5 days in the fridge or 1 month in the freezer.

If cooking from frozen, defrost overnight in the fridge. Reheat in a 200°C oven for about 20 minutes.

Baked Caprese Chicken

Ingredients

2 chicken breasts (about 500 g), butterflied into 4 pieces

½ teaspoon salt

½ teaspoon black pepper

4 handfuls baby spinach, shredded

3 garlic cloves, finely chopped

1 bunch basil, leaves picked

250 g mozzarella, thinly sliced

1 punnet cherry tomatoes

2 tablespoons olive oil

Method

1. Preheat the oven to 180°C.
2. Season the chicken with the salt and pepper. In a bowl, combine the spinach with the garlic and basil leaves. Divide the spinach mixture between each piece of chicken and top with a couple of slices of mozzarella. Roll the top half of the chicken over to encase the mixture.
3. Place the rolled chicken, seam side down, in a baking dish and top with more slices of mozzarella and 3–4 cherry tomatoes. Drizzle over the olive oil.
4. Bake for 20–25 minutes or until the chicken is tender and the cheese is bubbling and melted.

Serving Suggestion

Serve with boiled new potatoes and a rocket salad.

Storage & Reheating

The components of this simple meal can be kept separately in the fridge for the week. Only combine the ingredients on the day you wish to cook the dish.

Cool completely before chilling or freezing. The cooked chicken will keep for up to 1 week in the fridge or 2 months in the freezer.

To cook from frozen, defrost overnight in the fridge. Reheat, covered, in a 180°C oven until evenly heated through.

Marinated Salmon with Quinoa

Ingredients

4 cm piece ginger, grated
1 garlic clove, grated
2 tablespoons mirin
2 tablespoons low-sodium soy
    sauce
800 g salmon fillet, cut in 4

¾ cup quinoa
½ bunch kale, stalks removed and
    leaves finely shredded
juice of ½ lemon
1 tablespoon canola, sunflower or
    grapeseed oil

Method

1. Combine ginger, garlic, mirin and soy sauce in a small bowl. Place the salmon in a zip lock bag and add the marinade.

★ **At this point, the salmon can be frozen or kept uncooked in the fridge for up to 3 days.**

2. Cook the quinoa according to packet instructions then combine with the kale and lemon juice.

★ **At this point, the quinoa can be frozen or kept in the fridge for 5–7 days.**

3. Heat the oil in a non-stick frying or griddle pan over medium heat. Add the salmon, skin side down, and fry for 2–3 minutes on each side or until cooked through.

4. Serve with the quinoa and kale on the side.

Storage & Reheating

You can marinate and chill or freeze the uncooked salmon, or marinate, cook and then chill or freeze. The quinoa can also be chilled or frozen once it is cooked for up to 2 months. Uncooked salmon will keep for up to 3 months in the freezer. Cooked salmon will keep for 5–7 days in the fridge or 1 month in the freezer. To cook the uncooked salmon from frozen, defrost in zip lock bag overnight in the fridge then follow steps 3–4 to cook. To reheat cooked salmon from frozen, defrost overnight in the fridge, then follow steps 3–4 to cook. Defrost the quinoa overnight in the fridge and gently heat in a saucepan before serving.

Japanese-Style Steak Salad

Ingredients

4 cm piece ginger, grated
2 tablespoons low-sodium soy
    sauce
1 tablespoon mirin
½ teaspoon brown sugar
700 g eye fillet steak
1 head broccoli, florets chopped,
    stalk peeled and thinly sliced

1 large handful green beans,
    topped and tailed
2 handfuls baby spinach
2 cucumbers, cut into long batons
¼ red cabbage, finely shredded
1 tablespoon toasted sesame seeds

Dressing

1 tablespoon rice vinegar
1 teaspoon soy sauce

1 teaspoon mirin

Method

1. Combine the ginger with the soy sauce, mirin and brown sugar in a large bowl. Place the steak in the marinade and set aside in the fridge for at least an hour.

* **At this point, you can transfer the uncooked steak and the marinade to a zip lock bag and freeze.**

2. Blanch the broccoli and beans for 2 minutes in boiling water. Drain and transfer to a bowl.
3. Grill the steak in a hot griddle pan for 5–6 minutes on each side. Remove from the heat and set aside for 10 minutes.
4. Combine the dressing ingredients in a small bowl. Add the baby spinach, cucumber and shredded cabbage to the broccoli and beans.
5. Slice the steak into thin pieces and add to the salad. Pour over the prepared dressing and toasted sesame seeds and toss thoroughly to combine.

Storage & Reheating

The marinated steak will keep well in the fridge or freezer before cooking and can also be frozen once cooked and sliced. The salad components should stay in the fridge for last-minute preparation.

Uncooked steak will keep for up to 1 week in the fridge or 3 months in the freezer. Cooked steak will keep for up to 1 week in the fridge or 2 months in the freezer.

Defrost both the uncooked and cooked steak overnight in the fridge. Cooked steak can be added to the salad cold, or warmed briefly on the stovetop. Follow step 3 to cook the uncooked marinated steak.

Indian-Spiced Chicken & Cauliflower 'Rice'

Ingredients

2 garlic cloves, finely chopped

1 teaspoon ground cumin

1 teaspoon ground coriander

1 teaspoon garam masala

½ teaspoon turmeric

pinch of cayenne pepper

2 tablespoons olive oil

2 chicken breasts (about 500 g), butterflied into 4 pieces

1 cup beansprouts

Cauliflower Rice

1 cauliflower head, florets chopped

1 garlic clove, finely chopped

1 tablespoon rice vinegar

Method

1. In a large bowl, combine the garlic, spices and 1 tablespoon of oil and season with salt and pepper. Add the chicken and toss thoroughly to coat.

★ **At this point, the chicken can be transferred to a zip lock bag and frozen.**

2. To prepare the cauliflower rice, pulse the florets in a food processor or blender until they resemble rice grains.

3. Heat a large frying pan over medium heat and dry-fry the cauliflower, garlic and rice vinegar, stirring frequently, for 10 minutes or until the cauliflower has softened. Transfer the cauliflower rice to a bowl.

4. Rinse the frying pan and return to medium heat. Add 1 tablespoon of oil and fry the chicken for 2 minutes on each side or until cooked through. Serve the chicken on top of the cauliflower rice.

Storage & Reheating

The uncooked chicken will keep for up to 1 week in the fridge or up to 3 months in the freezer. Once cooked, the chicken will keep for 1 week in the fridge or up to 2 months in the freezer. Refrigerate the (uncooked) cauliflower rice for approximately 2 days. For best results, cooked cauliflower rice should be consumed same day as cooking.

Defrost the uncooked or cooked chicken overnight in the fridge. Follow step 4 to cook the chicken. Reheat the cooked chicken thoroughly in a pan, prior to making the cauliflower 'rice'. Follow step 3 to cook the cauliflower 'rice'.

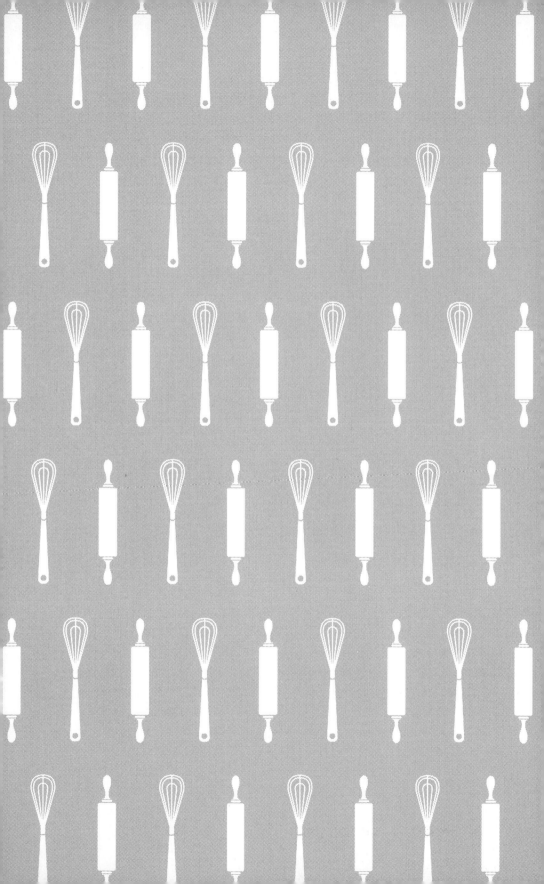

For Your Family & a Family in Need

For Your Family & a Family in Need

When a family you know hits Struggle Town, dropping a meal over lets that family know you care about them, that they are in your thoughts without the pressure of explanations on their part and gives them one less thing to think about and do.

And from the other side of the fence, how cared-for do we feel when a friend or an acquaintance drops over a home-cooked meal when we're sick, feeling a bit down or having a general rough time of it? We don't think anything can beat it!

This plan has been created so that you can cook enough for two families without blowing out your budget.

Menu

Vegetable Pizzas

Chicken, Bacon & Vegetable Pie

Slow-Cooked Chinese Beef Stew

Rich Bolognese Sauce

Pumpkin, Sweet Potato & Rosemary Soup

Sausage & Bean Hot-Pot

Potato, Cauliflower, Leek & Chorizo Gratin

Shopping List

Meat & Fish	Fruit & Veg	Dairy & Frozen
1.5 kg quality pork sausages 800 g beef mince 1.5 kg beef chuck steak 4 chorizo sausages 2 kg chicken breasts 12 rashers bacon	9 onions 3 heads garlic 4 cm piece ginger 8 large potatoes 2 large sweet potatoes 14 carrots 2 leeks 1 bunch celery 1 large butternut pumpkin 2 red capsicums 1 green capsicum 24 button mushrooms 1 head cauliflower 4 handfuls baby spinach 3 spring onions 1 bunch thyme 1 bunch rosemary 1 bunch coriander 1 bunch basil 1 bunch oregano	225 g plus 2 tbs butter 1 cup milk 185 ml cream 400 g mozzarella 250 g Swiss cheese 100 g parmesan 1 cup frozen peas

Tins, Jars & Dry Goods	Pantry Essentials	
5 x 400 g tins whole peeled tomatoes 3 x 400 g tins cannellini beans ½ cup pitted olives	olive oil canola, sunflower or grapeseed oil 3 litres vegetable stock 1.1 litres chicken stock 1.5 kg plain flour 4 tsp dry active yeast 3 tbs plus 1 tsp brown sugar 250 g jar tomato paste ¼ cup Shao Xing cooking wine (or dry sherry)	salt pepper 2 tbs mustard 3 tbs soy sauce 3 star anise 1 cinnamon stick

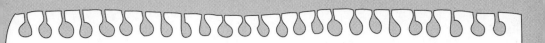

Serving Size

Each meal will feed approximately 2 families of 4 (8–10 serves)

Preparation time

3.5 hours

Equipment

Preparation: blender or food processor (optional), sharp knives, chopping boards suitable for vegetables and meat, kitchen scales, measuring cups and spoons, vegetable peeler, grater, mixing bowls in assorted sizes, rolling pin, whisk, mixing spoon.

Cooking: large, heavy-based frying pan, small, medium-sized and large saucepans, large ovenproof dish with lid, 2 baking dishes, (disposable aluminium baking dishes are handy when bulk cooking), 2 pie dishes.

Storage: zip lock bags, airtight containers suitable for freezing, foil.

Storage & Reheating

All the meals in this plan are freezer-friendly. We recommend that you first freeze all of your friend's meals and then deliver them within a couple of days. Alternatively, you can deliver them the day you have made them without freezing.

For your family, the meals in this plan can be refrigerated for up to 1 week, until the day you want to eat them.

Once-A-Week Cooking Preparation

	Total	Vegetable Pizzas	Chicken, Bacon & Vegetable Pie	Slow-Cooked Chinese Beef Stew
Doughs				
Pizza dough		prepare the dough and set aside to rest for 1½–2 hours	prepare the pastry and set aside in the fridge	
Fresh Produce				
Onions	9	1 thinly sliced	2 finely chopped	2 roughly chopped
Garlic	3	4 cloves, finely chopped	4 cloves, finely chopped	4 cloves, finely chopped
Ginger	4 cm piece			4 cm piece, finely chopped
Potatoes	8			
Sweet potatoes	2			
Carrots	14		4 finely diced	6 roughly diced
Leeks	2			
Celery	1		6 stalks, finely diced	
Butternut pumpkin	1			
Red capsicum	2	2 deseeded and thinly sliced		
Green capsicum	1	1 deseeded and thinly sliced		
Mushrooms	24	12 thinly sliced	12 thinly sliced	
Cauliflower	1			
Spring onions	3			3 tops finely sliced, ends roughly chopped
Thyme	1		4 sprigs, leaves picked	
Rosemary	1			
Coriander	1			roots washed and thinly sliced, leaves picked and finely chopped
Basil	1	1 bunch, leaves picked		
Oregano	1	1 bunch, leaves picked		

Rich Bolognese Sauce	Pumpkin, Sweet Potato & Rosemary Soup	Sausage & Bean Hot-Pot	Potato, Cauliflower, Leek & Chorizo Gratin
2 finely chopped	2 finely chopped		
8 cloves, finely chopped	5 cloves, finely chopped	4 cloves, finely chopped	6 cloves, peeled
			8 peeled and thinly sliced
	2 large, peeled and cut into 8 pieces each		
4 finely diced			
			2 thinly sliced
8 stalks, finely diced	5 finely diced		
	1 large, seeds removed and cut into large chunks		
			1 head, cut into florets, stalk thinly sliced
5 sprigs, leaves picked and finely chopped		6 sprigs, leaves picked and finely chopped	
5 sprigs, leaves picked and finely chopped	4 sprigs, leaves picked		3 sprigs, leaves picked

Once-A-Week Cooking Preparation

continued

	Total	Vegetable Pizzas	Chicken, Bacon & Vegetable Pie	Slow-Cooked Chinese Beef Stew
Cheese				
Mozzarella	400 g	400 g, grated		
Swiss cheese	250 g			
Parmesan	100 g			
Meat				
Chicken breasts	2 kg		2 kg, cut into 2–3 cm cubes	
Chorizo sausages	4			
Bacon	12		6 rashers, thinly sliced	
Beef chuck steak	1.5 kg			1.5 kg, cut into 2–3 cm pieces

Rich Bolognese Sauce	Pumpkin, Sweet Potato & Rosemary Soup	Sausage & Bean Hot-Pot	Potato, Cauliflower, Leek & Chorizo Gratin
			250 g, grated
100 g, grated			
			4 peeled and cut into ½ cm-thick pieces
6 rashers, finely chopped			

Once-A-Week Cooking Plan

1. Prepare the pizza dough for the **Vegetable Pizzas** and the pastry for the **Chicken, Bacon & Vegetable Pie**.

2. Preheat the oven to 180°C. Place 3 large saucepans on the stovetop for the **Chicken, Bacon & Vegetable Pie**, **Chinese Beef Stew** and **Rich Bolognese Sauce**.

3. Prepare the **Chicken, Bacon & Vegetable Pie** filling so it has time to cook and cool before filling the pastry case.

4. Prepare and cook **Slow-Cooked Chinese Beef Stew** as it has a long cooking time.

5. Make the **Rich Bolognese Sauce** and allow to simmer.

6. Roast the vegetables for the **Pumpkin, Sweet Potato & Rosemary Soup**.

7. Put together the **Potato, Cauliflower, Leek & Chorizo Gratin** and place in the oven.

8. Put together the **Sausage & Bean Hot-Pot** and allow to simmer for 30 minutes.

9. Finish off the **Pumpkin, Sweet Potato & Rosemary Soup**.

10. Once the dough has risen, put together the **Vegetable Pizzas**. If baking some of the pizzas, increase the oven temperature to 200°C. Bake or freeze as necessary.

11. Finally, roll out the pastry and form the cases for the **Chicken, Bacon & Vegetable Pie**. Fill with the cooled pie mixture and either freeze or bake.

12. Allow all cooked dishes to cool completely before chilling or freezing.

Vegetable Pizzas

Ingredients
Dough
1.1 kg plain flour, plus extra for dusting

4 teaspoons salt

4 tablespoons olive oil

4 teaspoons dry active yeast

740 ml warm water

Topping
1 tablespoon olive oil, plus extra for drizzling

4 garlic cloves, finely chopped

3 tablespoons tomato paste

1 x 400 g tin whole peeled tomatoes

1 teaspoon brown sugar

1 onion, thinly sliced

2 red capsicums, deseeded and thinly sliced

1 green capsicum, deseeded and thinly sliced

12 button mushrooms, thinly sliced

4 handfuls baby spinach

½ cup pitted olives

1 bunch basil, leaves picked, stalks discarded

1 bunch oregano, leaves picked, stalks discarded (or 4 tablespoons dried oregano)

400 g mozzarella, grated

Method
1. To make the dough, place the flour, salt and olive oil in the bowl of a stand mixer or large bowl.
2. In a separate jug or bowl, add the yeast to the warm water and set aside for 10 minutes until the mixture begins to froth. Pour into the flour and mix until a rough dough forms.
3. If you are using a stand mixer, knead the dough for 5 minutes. Alternatively, if you are making the dough by hand, scrape the dough onto a well-floured surface and knead for about 8–10 minutes.
4. Scrape the dough into a large lightly oiled bowl and cover with plastic wrap. Set aside for 1½–2 hours or until doubled in size.
5. Heat the olive oil in a small saucepan over medium heat. Add the garlic and sauté until translucent but not coloured. Add the tomato

paste and cook for 2 minutes. Add the whole peeled tomatoes and sugar and simmer for 8 minutes, or until the mixture has reduced by one-quarter. Remove from the heat and set aside to cool.

6. Tip the dough onto a well-floured surface and divide into 6 pieces. Roll each piece into a ball and then roll out into a large circle, about 1.5 cm thick. Place each dough circle on baking trays, pizza trays or whatever you have available.

7. Cover each pizza base with the sauce and top with the vegetables, olives, herbs and cheese (or whatever combination you like). Do not overload the pizzas with too many toppings as this prevents the bottom from crisping and leads to soggy pizza.

★ **At this point, the pizzas can be frozen (we recommend you freeze your friend's pizzas).**

8. Preheat the oven to 200°C.

9. Bake each pizza for about 20 minutes, until the toppings and cheese are hot and bubbling.

Serving Suggestion
Serve with a fresh green salad.

Storage & Reheating
Uncooked pizzas will keep for up to 2–3 months in the freezer or refrigerated for up to 5 days. Ensure pizzas are well wrapped before freezing or refrigerating. Allow the cooked pizzas to completely cool before chilling or freezing. They will keep for 5 days in the fridge or 2 months in the freezer.

If cooking from frozen, defrost on the kitchen bench for 1 hour before reheating in a 200°C oven, until the cheese is brown and bubbling on top. Add more cheese, if desired.

Chicken, Bacon & Vegetable Pie

Ingredients

2 kg chicken breasts, cut into 2–3 cm cubes

3 tablespoons plain flour

2 tablespoons oil

6 rashers fatty bacon, thinly sliced

4 carrots, finely diced

2 onions, finely chopped

6 celery stalks, finely diced

12 button mushrooms, thinly sliced

1 cup frozen peas

4 garlic cloves, finely chopped

4 thyme sprigs, leaves picked

60 ml cream

400 ml chicken stock

Shortcrust pastry

340 g plain flour, plus extra for dusting

1 teaspoon salt

225 g cold butter, diced

110 ml very cold water

Method

1. To make the pastry, combine the flour and salt in a large bowl. Rub the butter through the flour until the mixture resembles chunky breadcrumbs. Make a well and add the cold water. Mix to combine and form into a smooth, firm dough. Alternatively, you can make the dough in a stand mixer or food processor.

2. Wrap dough in plastic wrap and set aside in the fridge to chill for at least 1 hour.

3. Place the chicken and the flour in a large bowl and toss well to thoroughly coat the chicken.

4. Heat the oil in a large heavy-based saucepan over medium heat. Add the chicken and bacon and cook, stirring frequently, until the chicken browns. Add the vegetables and garlic and sauté for 10–15 minutes, or until the onion is translucent. Add the thyme, cream and chicken stock and bring to a simmer.

5. Allow to cook, uncovered, for 20–30 minutes, until the chicken is cooked through, the vegetables are tender and the sauce has reduced. Remove from the heat, and set aside to cool.

6. Preheat the oven to 180°C.
7. Cut the dough into 4 pieces. On a well-floured work surface, roll each piece out to a ½ cm-thick circle. Slide your hands under the dough and gently loosen it by moving your fingers. This encourages your dough to pre-shrink before you line your pie dish, so that it won't shrink in the oven. Roll out further if necessary, then line two 25 cm–30 cm pie dishes with 2 dough circles and trim any excess pastry.
8. Fill each base with the cooled chicken pie mixture. Do not exceed the height of the pastry. Cover the mixture with the remaining dough circles and trim the edges. Use a fork to seal the base and the top together. Cut an X in the centre of each pie top so steam can be released.

* At this point, the pie can be frozen.

9. Bake for 40–50 minutes or until the pastry is golden on top. Allow to cool for at least 10 minutes before serving.

Serving Suggestion
Serve with mashed potatoes and steamed vegetables.

Storage & Reheating
Uncooked pies will keep for up to 3 months in the freezer or a day in the fridge. Allow the cooked pies to cool completely before chilling or freezing. They will keep for 1 week in the fridge or 2 months in the freezer.

The uncooked pies can be cooked from frozen. Preheat the oven to 180°C. Brush the top of the frozen pie with a little milk or lightly beaten egg and cook for around 40 minutes or until hot all the way through. Cover with foil if the pastry is browning too quickly.

If reheating a cooked pie from frozen, defrost overnight in the fridge. Preheat the oven to 180°C and cover the pie with foil. Bake until heated through evenly.

Slow-Cooked Chinese Beef Stew

Shao Xing cooking wine can be found in Asian grocery stores. You can replace it with dry sherry

Ingredients

2 tablespoons neutral oil such as rice bran oil

1.5 kg beef chuck steak, cut into 2–3 cm pieces

6 carrots, roughly diced

2 onions, roughly chopped

4 garlic cloves, finely chopped

1 x 4 cm piece ginger, finely chopped

3 spring onions, ends roughly chopped, tops finely sliced, for garnish

1 bunch coriander, roots washed and thinly sliced, leaves picked and finely chopped, for garnish

3 star anise

1 cinnamon stick

3 tablespoons soy sauce

1 tablespoon brown sugar

¼ cup Shao Xing cooking wine (or dry sherry)

400 ml chicken stock

½ teaspoon pepper

½ teaspoon salt

Method

1. Preheat the oven to 150°C.
2. Heat the oil in a large casserole dish or Dutch oven over high heat. Add the beef in batches and brown on all sides. (Cooking in several batches prevents overcrowding in the dish and allows the meat to caramelise properly, for maximum flavour.)
3. Return all of the beef to the casserole dish and add the carrot, onion, garlic and ginger. Stir to combine and cook for 10 minutes. Add the coriander root and spring onion ends along with the spices, soy sauce, brown sugar, Shao Xing wine, stock, seasoning and 1 cup water. Bring to the boil, cover and remove from the heat.
4. Place in the preheated oven and cook, covered, for 1½ hours or until the sauce has reduced and beef is very tender and can be pulled apart. Season to taste again and garnish with the coriander leaves and spring onion tops.

Serving Suggestion

Serve the stew with steamed jasmine rice on the side.

Storage & Reheating

Allow to cool completely before decanting into containers and freezing. This stew will keep for 1 week in the fridge or 2 months in the freezer.

To cook from frozen, defrost overnight in fridge. Reheat thoroughly in a microwave or saucepan.

Rich Bolognese Sauce

Ingredients

2 tablespoons olive oil

2 onions, finely chopped

4 carrots, finely diced

8 celery stalks, finely diced

8 garlic cloves, finely chopped

800 g beef mince

4 tablespoons tomato paste

5 rosemary sprigs, leaves picked and finely chopped

5 thyme sprigs, leaves picked and finely chopped

6 rashers bacon, finely chopped

2 x 400 g tins whole peeled tomatoes

1 cup chicken stock

100 g parmesan, grated

Method

1. Heat the olive oil in a large, heavy-based saucepan over medium heat. Add the vegetables, bacon and garlic and sauté until tender, about 10–15 minutes. Add the mince and brown while breaking it up with a wooden spoon. Add the tomato paste to one side of the pan and cook off for 2 minutes before stirring through the meat and vegetables. Add the herbs, tinned tomatoes and stock and bring to a simmer.

2. Cook, covered, over a low heat for 1¼–1½ hours until the sauce thickens.

3. Stir through the parmesan at the end and season, to taste.

Serving Suggestion

Spoon Bolognese over al dente spaghetti and sprinkle with some grated parmesan.

Storage & Reheating

Allow to cool completely before chilling or freezing. The bolognese will keep for up to 1 week in the fridge or 3 months in the freezer.

To cook from frozen, defrost overnight in fridge. Reheat thoroughly in a microwave or saucepan.

Pumpkin, Sweet Potato & Rosemary Soup

Ingredients

1 large butternut pumpkin, seeds removed and cut into large chunks

2 large sweet potatoes, peeled and cut into 8 pieces each

2 tablespoons olive oil

2 onions, finely chopped

5 celery stalks, finely diced

5 garlic cloves, finely chopped

4 rosemary sprigs, leaves picked

3 litres vegetable stock

Method

1. Preheat the oven to 200°C.
2. Place the pumpkin and sweet potato in a large roasting tin, toss through 1 tablespoon oil and roast until tender, about 30 minutes.
3. Heat the remaining oil in a large heavy-based saucepan over medium heat. Sauté the onion, celery and garlic for about 10 minutes or until the onion is translucent.
4. Peel the skin from the pumpkin and add the flesh to the onion mixture along with the sweet potato. Add the rosemary leaves and stock and bring to the boil.
5. Reduce the heat to low and simmer for 30–40 minutes or until the vegetables are very tender and the flavours have infused.
6. If you do not have a blender or food processor, cook the vegetables until they can be mashed into a chunky soup. Otherwise, process the soup in batches and season with salt and pepper, to taste.

Serving Suggestion

Serve the soup with crusty bread on the side for dipping.

Storage & Reheating

Allow the soup to cool completely before dividing among containers and chilling or freezing. This meal will keep for 1 week in the fridge or 3 months in the freezer.

To cook from frozen, defrost overnight in the fridge. Reheat thoroughly in a microwave or saucepan.

Sausage & Bean Hot-Pot

Ingredients

2 tablespoons olive oil

1.5 kg quality pork sausages

4 garlic cloves, finely chopped

2 x 400 g tins whole peeled
   tomatoes

2 tablespoons mustard (Dijon or
   wholegrain)

2 tablespoons brown sugar

6 thyme sprigs, leaves picked and
   finely chopped

3 x 400 g tins cannellini beans,
   rinsed and drained

Method

1. Heat the oil in a large heavy-based frying pan over medium heat.
   Fry the sausages for about 5 minutes on each side or until brown.
   Add the garlic and stir until it starts to colour. Add the tinned
   tomatoes, mustard, sugar and cannellini beans and stir to combine.
2. Bring to a simmer, cover and cook for 30 minutes. Season with salt
   and pepper, to taste.

Serving Suggestion

This hot-pot is fantastic served with crusty bread and a green salad on
the side.

Storage & Reheating

Allow the hot-pot to cool completely before dividing between two
containers and chilling or freezing. It will keep for up to 1 week in the
fridge or 2 months in the freezer.

To cook from frozen, defrost overnight in the fridge. Reheat
thoroughly in a microwave or saucepan.

Potato, Cauliflower, Leek & Chorizo Gratin

Ingredients

2 tablespoons butter, plus extra for greasing

½ cup cream

1 cup milk

3 rosemary sprigs, leaves picked

6 garlic cloves, peeled

8 large potatoes, peeled and thinly sliced

1 head cauliflower, cut into florets, stalk thinly sliced

2 leeks, thinly sliced

4 chorizo sausages, peeled and cut into ½ cm-thick pieces

250 g Swiss cheese, grated

Method

1. Preheat the oven to 180°C. Generously grease two ceramic baking dishes.
2. Place the butter, cream, milk, rosemary and peeled garlic in a small saucepan and bring just to the boil. Reduce the heat to very low and cook for 10 minutes. Discard the garlic. Set aside.
3. Divide the potato slices evenly between the baking dishes, then add a layer of cauliflower, the sliced leek and chorizo. Pour the infused milk and cream mixture over the vegetables and sprinkle the grated cheese over the top.
4. Bake for 40 minutes or until the top is golden and bubbling.

Serving Suggestion

Serve on a bed of baby spinach.

Storage & Reheating

Allow to cool completely before chilling or freezing. The gratin will keep for 1 week in the fridge but given the large quantity of cream and milk we don't recommend freezing this meal. To reheat from refrigeration cover with foil and bake at 180°C for about 30 minutes. Remove the foil for the last 5–10 minutes of cooking.

A Whole Month's Worth of Toddler Meals!

A Whole Month's Worth of Toddler Meals!

This one was always going to be tricky! Toddlers are at that Throw-ALL-The-Foods-On-The-Floor stage, so cooking for them can be a dispiriting experience.

Here is a plan of wholesome and tasty meals that can be easily frozen in quick-to-defrost portions.

If you are encouraging your toddler to eat the same meals as the rest of the family – great! But, having these meals cooked up as a back-up plan when they decide that they just cannot and will not eat what you are cooking for everyone will be a lifesaver.

In terms of serving suggestions, you will know what your child will prefer to eat with each of these meals.

Menu

Beef with Egg Noodles

Veggie-Filled Bolognese

Child-Friendly Fish Pie

Soft Chicken Rice

Chicken Meatballs

Bacon & Pea Frittata

Fish Fingers

Shopping List

Meat & Fish	Fruit & Veg	Dairy & Frozen
400 g salmon fillet 600 g firm white fish 400 g beef rump or blade 500 g beef mince 250 g chicken breasts 500 g chicken mince 150 g ham	2 onions 2 heads garlic 2 cm piece ginger 1 kg potatoes 2 celery stalks 3 carrots 2 red capsicums 3 handfuls baby spinach 1 bunch spring onions 4 thyme sprigs 1 bunch parsley 1 bunch chives 1 apple 1 lemon	200 g tasty cheese 35 g butter 550 ml milk 9 eggs 2 cups frozen peas

Tins, Jars & Dry Goods	Pantry Essentials	Other Ingredients

2 x 400 g tins crushed
    tomatoes
300 g breadcrumbs
1 cup small pasta
1 cup jasmine rice
	olive oil
	oil, for frying
	canola, sunflower or
	    grapeseed oil
	125 g plain flour
	375 ml chicken stock
	3 tbs tomato paste
	1 tsp sugar
	salt
	pepper
	2 tsp mustard
	2 tsp Worcestershire
	    sauce
	2 tbs soy sauce
	2 tbs oyster sauce
	1 tsp sweet paprika
		500 g fresh thin egg
		    noodles

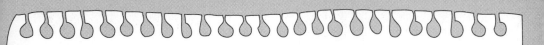

Serving Size
Each recipe makes approximately 6–10 serves

Preparation time
2.5 hours

Equipment
Preparation: grater, sharp knives, chopping boards, measuring spoons and cups, kitchen scales, rolling pin, food processor, potato musher, citrus zester and juicer, rice cooker (optional), edged baking sheet, large zip lock bag (optional).

Cooking: oven-proof casserole or Dutch oven, heavy-based saucepan or wok, small saucepan, large heavy-based frying pan, oven-proof dish.

Storage: zip lock bags, airtight containers suitable for freezing, foil.

Storage & Reheating
All of these meals are freezer-friendly and will keep for 1–2 months in the freezer. Each meal should be portioned according to the instructions in the individual recipes or according to how much your child will eat.

As the portions are toddler-sized, you can defrost them quickly on the day you wish to cook them.

The Fish Fingers can be cooked from frozen, while the Child-Friendly Fish Pie, Veggie-Filled Bolognese, Chicken Meatballs, Soft Chicken Rice and Beef with Egg Noodles require at least 1 hour to defrost, so that blast-heating in a saucepan or microwave does not destroy the texture or flavour.

Because the intention is to prepare a mixture of meals that will appeal to your toddler, it is recommended that you portion and freeze these meals so that every day can be different.

Once-A-Week Preparation

	Total	Beef with Egg Noodles	Veggie-filled Bolognese	Child-Friendly Fish Pie
Fresh Produce				
Onions	2		1 finely chopped	
Garlic	2	2 cloves, finely chopped	2 cloves, finely chopped	
Ginger	2 cm piece	1 cm piece, finely chopped		
Potatoes	1 kg			1 kg, peeled and diced
Celery	2		2 stalks, finely chopped	
Carrots	3	1 julienned	2 grated	
Capsicums	2	1 julienned	1 finely chopped	
Spring onions	1	3 thinly sliced		4 thinly sliced
Thyme	1			
Parsley	1			
Chives	1			1 bunch, finely chopped
Apple	1		1 grated	
Lemon	1			
Cheese				
Tasty cheese	200 g			100 g, grated
Meat & Fish				
Salmon	400 g			400 g, diced (ensure there are no bones)
Firm white fish	600 g			
Beef rump or blade	400 g	400 g, thinly sliced		
Chicken breast	250 g			
Ham	150 g			

Soft Chicken Rice	Chicken Meatballs	Bacon & Pea Frittata	Fish Fingers
		1 finely chopped	
5 cloves, finely chopped	3 cloves, finely chopped		
1 cm piece, finely chopped			
3 thinly sliced			
	4 sprigs, leaves picked and finely chopped		
		½ bunch, finely chopped	½ bunch, finely chopped
	1 zested		
		100 g, grated	
			600 g, cut into long strips
250 g, cut into 1 cm-thick slices			
		150 g, diced	

Once-A-Week Cooking Plan

1. Preheat the oven to 180°C. Boil the kettle for the noodles in the **Beef with Egg Noodles**.

2. Boil the potatoes for the **Child-Friendly Fish Pie**.

3. Prepare the **Veggie-Filled Bolognese Sauce** and simmer for 45 minutes.

4. Next, prepare the **Child-Friendly Fish Pie** and bake.

5. Put together the **Soft Chicken Rice** and cook.

6. Prepare the **Chicken Meatballs** mixture. Set a large shallow frying pan over medium heat and fry the meatballs while the other dishes bake or simmer.

7. Prepare and cook the **Beef with Egg Noodles**.

8. Make the **Bacon & Pea Frittata**. Place in the oven to brown for 5 minutes.

9. Finally, set up a production line of flour, egg mixture and breadcrumbs for the **Fish Fingers**. Fry these or freeze them for frying from frozen.

10. Allow all dishes to cool completely before dividing into portions and chilling or freezing.

Beef with Egg Noodles

Ingredients

500 g fresh thin egg noodles

400 g beef rump or blade, thinly sliced

2 garlic cloves, finely chopped

1 cm piece ginger, finely chopped

1 tablespoon soy sauce

1 teaspoon sugar

2 tablespoons oyster sauce

2 tablespoons canola, sunflower or grapeseed oil

1 carrot, julienned

1 red capsicum, julienned

3 spring onions, thinly sliced

1 handful baby spinach

Method

1. Place the noodles in a heat-proof bowl and pour over enough boiling water to submerge the noodles. Leave for 2 minutes before loosening the noodles with a fork. Drain and set aside.

2. In a large bowl, combine the beef with the garlic, ginger, soy sauce, sugar and oyster sauce.

3. Heat the oil in a large heavy-based frying pan or wok over high heat. Add the carrot and capsicum and cook, stirring frequently, for 5–7 minutes or until slightly softened. Add the beef and fry until just tender. Add the spring onion and softened noodles and toss to combine. Throw in the baby spinach and stir until it wilts. Remove from the heat and set aside to cool.

Storing & Reheating

Allow to cool completely before dividing into portions and chilling or freezing. This dish will keep for 3 days in the fridge or 1 month in the freezer.

For best results, allow to defrost for a minimum of 1 hour before reheating. Heat in a hot wok until evenly warmed through and any liquid released from defrosting has evaporated.

Veggie-Filled Bolognese

Ingredients

2 tablespoons olive oil
1 onion, finely chopped
2 garlic cloves, finely chopped
2 celery stalks, finely chopped
1 red capsicum, finely chopped
2 carrots, grated

1 apple, grated
2 handfuls baby spinach
500 g beef mince
3 tablespoons tomato paste
1 cup chicken stock
2 x 400 g tins crushed tomatoes

Method

1. Heat 1 tablespoon of the olive oil in a large heavy-based casserole or Dutch oven. Add the onion, garlic, celery and red capsicum and sauté until the onion is translucent. Add the carrot, apple and spinach and cook for a further 10 minutes. (Tip: If your toddler is particularly picky about vegetables, you can purée them at this point in a blender or food processor before returning them to the pan.)
2. Add the beef mince and stir to combine, breaking up any lumps with the back of a wooden spoon. Cook for at least 10 minutes until cooked through. Add the tomato paste and stir to combine. Allow to cook out for a few minutes.
3. Add the stock and tinned tomatoes and simmer, stirring occasionally, for 35–45 minutes or until the sauce has thickened. Season to taste and set aside to cool.

Serving Suggestion

Spoon Bolognese over al dente spaghetti and sprinkle with some grated parmesan.

Storage & Reheating

Allow to cool completely before dividing into individual portions and chilling or freezing. The bolognese will keep for up to 1 week in the fridge or 3 months in the freezer.

For best results, allow to defrost for a minimum of 1 hour before reheating. Reheat thoroughly in microwave or saucepan.

Child-Friendly Fish Pie

Ingredients

1 kg potatoes, peeled and diced

2 cups milk

35 g butter plus a knob of butter
for the mash

25 g plain flour

4 spring onions, thinly sliced

400 g salmon, diced and double-
checked for bones

1 bunch chives, finely chopped

1 cup frozen peas

1 teaspoon mild mustard (as per
your child's taste)

100 g tasty cheese, grated

Method

1. Preheat the oven to 180°C. Lightly grease a ceramic baking dish.
2. Boil the potatoes in a large saucepan of salted water until tender. Drain, transfer to a large bowl and mash with 200 ml milk (add more or less according to your child's preferred consistency) and a knob of the butter. Set aside.
3. Using the same saucepan, melt the butter then add the flour and spring onion. Stir over medium heat until the mixture resembles wet sand. Whisk in 300 ml of milk and bring to the boil. Whisk continuously for 3–4 minutes or until the béchamel has thickened. Season with salt and pepper, to taste.
4. Add the salmon, chives, peas, mustard and half of the cheese. Stir to combine. Pour the fish mixture into the baking dish (or divide among individual ramekins if you prefer to cook each serve as needed). Spoon the mash over the top and sprinkle with the remaining cheese.
5. Bake for 25–30 minutes or until golden.

Storage & Reheating

All to cool completely before dividing into portions and chilling or freezing. The fish pie will keep uncooked in the fridge for up to 3 days or 1 week once cooked. It will keep uncooked or cooked for up to 2 months in the freezer.

For best results, defrost for a minimum of 1 hour before cooking or reheating. Preheat the oven to 180°C and bake for 45 minutes or until the pie is heated all the way through.

Soft Chicken Rice

Ingredients

1 cup jasmine rice
½ cup chicken stock
5 garlic cloves, finely chopped
1 cm piece ginger, finely chopped

250 g chicken breast, cut into 1 cm-thick slices
3 spring onions, thinly sliced
soy sauce, to taste

Method

1. Place the rice, stock, garlic, ginger and 1 cup water in a medium-sized saucepan or a rice cooker. Add the chicken, bring to a simmer then reduce the heat to low and cook, covered, for 30 minutes.
2. At the end of cooking, top with the spring onion and season with soy sauce, to taste.

Storage & Reheating

Allow to cool completely before dividing into individual portions and chilling or freezing. The chicken rice will keep for up to 5 days in the fridge or 1 month in the freezer.

For best results, allow to defrost for a minimum of 1 hour before reheating. Reheat in a microwave or on the stovetop until evenly heated through, adding more liquid if necessary.

Chicken Meatballs

Ingredients

500 g chicken mince

3 garlic cloves, finely chopped

4 thyme sprigs, leaves picked and finely chopped

zest of 1 lemon

1 egg

100 g breadcrumbs

1 teaspoon sweet paprika

2 teaspoons Worcestershire sauce

1 teaspoon mild mustard (as per your child's taste)

1 teaspoon salt

½ teaspoon pepper

2 tablespoons canola, sunflower or grapeseed oil

Method

1. Combine all of the ingredients except the oil in a large bowl. Form the mixture into 30–40 meatballs.

★ **At this point, the meatballs can be frozen in individual portions.**

2. Heat the oil in a large heavy-based frying pan over medium–high heat. Fry the meatballs, in batches, for 3 minutes on each side. Drain on paper towel while you cook the remaining meatballs. Alternatively, you can poach the meatballs in simmering water.

Serving Suggestion

Serve meatballs with steamed broccoli and sprinkle with grated cheese.

Storage & Reheating

Uncooked meatballs will keep for 1 week in the fridge or 3 months in the freezer. Allow the cooked meatballs to cool completely before chilling or freezing. They will keep for up to 1 week in the fridge or 2 months in the freezer.

Defrost uncooked meatballs in the fridge overnight then follow the recipe from step 2. Defrost cooked meatballs overnight in the fridge then reheat thoroughly in the oven or microwave before serving.

Bacon & Pea Frittata

Ingredients

6 eggs

150 g sliced ham, diced

100 g tasty cheese, grated

1 cup frozen peas

½ bunch parsley, finely chopped

½ teaspoon salt

¼ teaspoon pepper

1 cup small pasta

1 tablespoon olive oil

1 onion, finely chopped

Method

1. Preheat the oven to 180°C or heat your grill to high.
2. Beat the eggs in a bowl and season with salt and pepper. Add the ham, cheese, peas, parsley and seasoning.
3. Cook the pasta in salted boiling water until al dente. Drain and set aside.
4. Heat the olive oil in an ovenproof pan or skillet over medium heat. Add the onion and cook until translucent, about 5–8 minutes. Pour in the egg mixture and cook over low heat for 8 minutes or until nearly set. To cook the egg evenly, tilt the pan and draw the frittata edges in to leave room for the runny mixture to pour into the space left behind.
5. To finish, place the pan in the oven or under the grill for 5 minutes to brown and cook the top.

Storage & Reheating

Allow to cool completely before cutting into individual serves and chilling or freezing. The frittata will keep for up to 3 days in the fridge or 1 month in the freezer.

For best results, allow to defrost for a minimum of 1 hour before reheating. The frittata can be reheated in the microwave or in a 180°C oven, covered with foil and placed on a baking tray, for 30 minutes. Alternatively, eat cold once defrosted.

Fish Fingers

Ingredients

100 g plain flour
50 ml milk
2 eggs
200 g breadcrumbs
½ bunch parsley, finely chopped

1 teaspoon salt
½ teaspoon pepper
600 g firm white fish fillets,
   cut into long strips
200 ml oil for frying

Method

1. Place the flour, milk and eggs, and breadcrumbs into three bowls.
2. Beat the eggs with the milk.
3. Add the parsley to the breadcrumbs and mix. Season with the salt and pepper.
4. Coat each fish finger firstly with flour, then dip into the egg mixture, allowing any excess to drip off. Finally, coat the fish in breadcrumbs, pressing gently to adhere.
5. Heat the oil in a heavy-based frying pan until it reaches 180°C. You can test the temperature of the oil by dropping in a cube of bread. If it turns completely golden brown in 15 seconds, the oil is ready.
6. Fry about 3–4 fish fingers at a time for 3 minutes on each side. Drain on paper towel and repeat with the remaining fish.

Serving Suggestion

Serve with peas or steamed vegetables.

Storage & Reheating

Allow cooked fish fingers to cool completely before chilling or freezing. They will keep for up to 2 days in the fridge or 2 months in the freezer.

Cooked fish fingers can be reheated from frozen. Preheat the oven to 220°C, lightly grease a baking sheet and ensure the fish fingers are spread evenly and cook for 20 minutes or until heated all the way through. Turn the fingers halfway through reheating to ensure even cooking and golden brown on both sides.

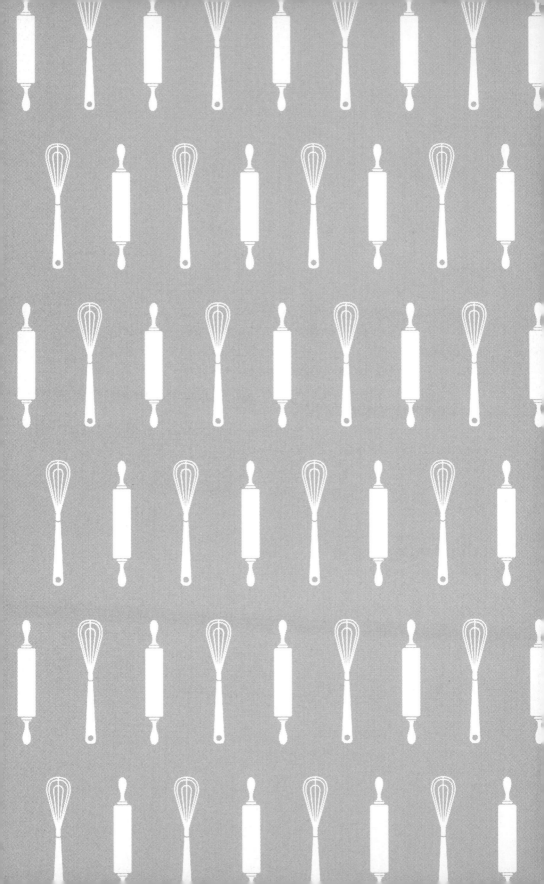

Budget Meat Menu

Budget Meat Menu

You don't need to spend a fortune on meat to create meals your family will love. When cooked properly, the cheaper, often overlooked cuts of meat develop flavour beautifully and cook to create tender, mouth-watering meals, for a fraction of the price.

MamaBaker Elsie says:

> "This plan is great for us. As a family on a strict food budget, I can't spend a fortune on meat every week. I time my shopping to coincide with when my local butcher reduces their prices every Sunday afternoon and then I end up saving even more! The pulled pork is the favourite meal from this plan for my family, although all the meals have been eaten with no complaint!"

Budget meat cuts guide

Beef: chuck, oyster blade, bolar blade, silverside, shank or shin, brisket, flank, leg and top rump
Lamb: shoulder, neck, breast, rump and shank
Pork: neck, shoulder, spare rib, chump, cheek and belly (in recent times this cut has become fashionable and, therefore, more expensive).
Chicken: drumsticks and wings.

Menu

Osso Bucco with Quick Gremolata

Lamb Shank Ragù

Beef Stew

Pulled Pork

Beef Noodle Stir-Fry

One-Tray Chicken Drumsticks

Chicken Wing Soup

Shopping List

Meat & Fish	Fruit & Veg	Dairy & Frozen
1.5 kg beef bolar blade 3 kg pork shoulder 1 kg chicken drumsticks 1 kg chicken wings 1.5 kg osso bucco 2 kg lamb shanks	5 onions 2 heads garlic 4 cm piece ginger 6 potatoes 15 carrots 2 parsnips or turnips 2 bunches celery 1 red capsicum 10 button mushrooms ¼ white cabbage 2 bunches spring onions 1 bunch coriander 1 bunch sage 1 bunch thyme 1 bunch rosemary 2 bunches parsley 4 lemons	1 cup frozen peas 350 g cold butter 1 egg

Tins, Jars & Dry Goods	Pantry Essentials	Other Ingredients
2 x 400 g tins whole peeled tomatoes 1 x 400 g tin crushed tomatoes ¾ cup basmati rice ½ cup pearl barley sesame seeds (optional)	canola, sunflower or grapeseed oil olive oil 1.25 litres beef stock 2 litres chicken stock 3 tbs tomato paste 2½ tbs brown sugar 2 tbs honey salt pepper 2 tbs soy sauce 2 tsp sesame oil 3 tbs oyster sauce 455 g plain flour, plus extra for dusting 1 tbs smoked paprika 4 star anise	1 cup wine 2 x 500 g pack Hokkien-style yellow noodles

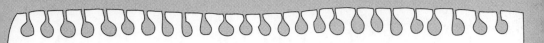

Serving Size
Each meal serves a family of 4 (approximately)

Preparation time
4.5 hours

Equipment
Preparation: sharp knives, chopping boards suitable for vegetables and fruit, meat and fish, kitchen scales, measuring cups and spoons, vegetable peeler, grater, food processor or blender, sealed container, large bowls.
Cooking: large heavy-based saucepan, frying pan or wok, large heavy-based casserole dishes or Dutch ovens with lids, large heavy-based baking dishes, stockpot, two 23 cm pie dishes.
Storage: airtight containers suitable for freezing, zip lock bag, foil.

Storage & Reheating
Please refer to individual recipes for storage and heating instructions.

Once-A-Week Cooking Preparation

	Total	Osso Bucco with Quick Gremolata	Lamb Shank Ragù	Beef Stew
Fresh Produce				
Onions	5	2 finely chopped	1 finely chopped	1 chopped
Garlic	2	7 cloves, finely chopped	4 cloves, finely chopped	3 cloves, finely chopped
Ginger	4 cm piece			
Potatoes	6			
Carrots	15		3 finely diced	3 diced
Parsnips or turnips	2			2 diced
Celery	2		5 stalks, finey diced	4 stalks, diced
Capsicums	1			
Button mushrooms	10			10 quartered
White cabbage	¼			
Spring onions	2			
Coriander	1			
Sage	1	3 sprigs, leaves picked		
Thyme	1	3 sprigs, leaves picked	2 sprigs, leaves picked	4 sprigs, leaves picked and finely chopped
Rosemary	1	2 sprigs, leaves picked	2 sprigs, leaves picked	4 sprigs, leaves picked and finely chopped
Parsley	2	1 bunch, finely chopped	1 bunch, finely chopped	
Lemon	4	1 zested	1 zested	
Meat				
Beef bolar blade	1.8 kg			1.5 kg cut into 3 cm dice

Beef Noodle Stir-Fry	One-Tray Chicken Drumsticks	Chicken Wing Soup
		1 chopped
3 cloves, finely chopped	3 cloves, finely chopped	5 cloves, smashed
		4 cm piece, thinly sliced
	6 cut into 8–10 chunks each	
2 julienned	4 cut into 8–10 chunks	3 diced
		4 stalks, diced
1 julienned		
		¼ finely shredded
1 bunch, tops cut into 4 cm-long pieces, ends discarded		3 tops thinly sliced, ends reserved
		1 bunch, roots washed and reserved, leaves roughly chopped
	4 sprigs, leaves picked	
	2 zested and thinly sliced	
300 g, thinly sliced		

Once-A-Week Cooking Plan

1. Preheat the oven to 150°C. Place two large heavy-based casserole dishes on the stovetop for the **Osso Bucco with Quick Gremolata** and **Lamb Shank Ragù**, and a large lidded saucepan for the **Beef Stew**.

2. Prepare the pork shoulder for the **Pulled Pork** and begin to slow cook.

3. Make the **Osso Bucco with Quick Gremolata**. As the oven is already at the correct temperature, this can be cooked alongside the **Pulled Pork**.

4. Brown the lamb shanks for the **Lamb Shank Ragù** and continue cooking.

5. Prepare and cook the **Beef Stew** filling. In the final hour of cooking, prepare the pie pastry. Assemble pies and bake.

6. Marinate the beef for the **Beef Noodle Stir-Fry**.

7. Prepare the chicken for the **One-Tray Chicken Drumsticks**.

8. Make the **Chicken Wing Soup** stock.

9. When the **Pulled Pork** and **Osso Bucco with Quick Gremolata** have finished cooking, bake the **One-Tray Chicken Drumsticks**.

10. Finish the **Chicken Wing Soup**.

11. Allow all dishes to cool completely before chilling or freezing. Decant the meals into airtight containers or zip lock bags to save space. Wrap pies well before freezing or refrigerating.

Osso Bucco with Quick Gremolata

Ingredients

4 tablespoons olive oil

1.5 kg osso bucco (about 4–6 pieces)

2 onions, finely chopped

4 garlic cloves, finely chopped

3 thyme sprigs, leaves picked

3 sage sprigs, leaves picked

2 rosemary sprigs, leaves picked

1 cup red or white wine

2 x 400 g tins whole peeled tomatoes

1 cup beef stock

Quick Gremolata

3 garlic cloves, finely chopped

1 bunch parsley, finely chopped

zest of 1 lemon

Method

1. Preheat the oven to 150°C. Season the osso bucco well on both sides.
2. Place a large heavy-based casserole dish or Dutch oven over medium–high heat and add 3 tablespoons of the olive oil. Add the osso bucco and brown the meat on both sides. Remove from the dish and set aside.
3. Reduce the heat to medium. Add the remaining olive oil along with the onion, garlic and herbs. Cook for 5–7 minutes until the onion is translucent. Return the heat to high and add the wine, stirring to combine. Cook until the liquid has reduced and you can no longer smell the alcohol, about 5 minutes. Add the tomatoes and stock and bring to the boil before reducing to a simmer.
4. Return the osso bucco to the dish and season the sauce, to taste. Cover with a lid and put the dish in the oven for 2–3 hours or until the meat is falling off the bone.
5. To make the gremolata, combine all of the ingredients in a small bowl.
6. Garnish the Osso Bucco with the gremolata and allow the meat to rest for 5 minutes before serving.

Serving Suggestion

Serve the Osso Bucco alongside mashed potato and a green salad.

Storage & Reheating

Allow to cool completely before chilling or freezing. This dish will keep for up to 1 week in the fridge or 2 months in the freezer.

To cook from frozen, defrost overnight in the fridge. Reheat thoroughly in a microwave or saucepan.

Lamb Shank Ragù

Ingredients

2 tablespoons canola, sunflower or grapeseed oil

2 kg lamb shanks

1 onion, finely chopped

5 celery stalks, finely diced

3 carrots, finely diced

4 garlic cloves, finely chopped

2 rosemary sprigs, leaves picked

2 thyme sprigs, leaves picked

1 x 400 g tin crushed tomatoes

½ teaspoon salt

½ cup pearl barley

1 bunch parsley, finely chopped

zest of 1 lemon

Method

1. Preheat the oven to 160°C.
2. Heat the oil in a large heavy-based casserole dish or Dutch oven over medium heat. Add the lamb shanks and brown on all sides. Remove from the dish and set aside.
3. Add the vegetables, ¾ of the garlic, rosemary and thyme to the dish and sauté until the onion is translucent.
4. Return the shanks to the dish and top with the crushed tomatoes, 1.5 litres water, the salt and some freshly ground pepper. Pop the lid on and place in the oven for 3–4 hours or until the meat is falling off the bone.
5. At the end of the cooking time, add the pearl barley and 1 cup water and stir to combine. Return to the oven and cook for a further 20 minutes or until the pearl barley is tender.
6. Combine the parsley, remaining garlic and lemon zest in a small bowl. Season the ragù then garnish with the parsley mixture and serve.

Serving Suggestion

Serve with creamy mashed potatoes.

Storage & Reheating

Allow to cool completely before chilling or freezing. The ragù will keep for 1 week in the fridge or up to 3 months in the freezer.

To cook from frozen, defrost overnight in the fridge. Reheat thoroughly in a microwave or saucepan.

Beef Stew

This recipe will yield two family-sized pies.

Ingredients

2 tablespoons canola, sunflower, or grapeseed oil

1.5 kg beef bolar blade, trimmed and cut into 3 cm dice

3 carrots, diced

4 celery stalks, diced

2 parsnips or turnips, diced

1 onion, chopped

3 garlic cloves, finely chopped

3 tablespoons tomato paste

4 rosemary sprigs, leaves picked and finely chopped

4 thyme sprigs, leaves picked and finely chopped

10 button mushrooms, quartered

1 cup frozen peas

1 litre beef stock

1½ teaspoons salt

Shortcrust pastry

455 g plain flour, plus extra for dusting

1 teaspoon salt

300 g cold butter, diced

150 ml very cold water

1 egg, beaten

sesame seeds (optional)

Method

1. Heat the oil in a large heavy-based saucepan over medium heat. Add the beef and brown on all sides. Remove from the saucepan and set aside.
2. Add the carrot, celery, parsnip or turnip, onion and garlic to the saucepan and sauté, stirring frequently, until the onion is translucent.
3. Return the beef to the saucepan and add the tomato paste. Allow the paste to cook off for a few minutes, then add the rosemary and thyme. Add the mushrooms, frozen peas, beef stock, salt and some black pepper.
4. Bring to a simmer and cook over low–medium heat for 2–3 hours until the beef is very tender. Stir occasionally to ensure that the stew is not catching on the bottom of the pan. The sauce should be reduced to just cover the beef and vegetables. Taste the stew and

season again if necessary. Transfer to a large dish and set aside to cool in the fridge.

5. Meanwhile, make the pastry. Combine the flour and salt in a large bowl. Rub the butter through the flour until the mixture resembles chunky breadcrumbs. Make a well and add the cold water. Mix to combine and form into a smooth, firm dough.

6. Wrap in plastic wrap and set aside in the fridge to chill for at least 1 hour. Alternatively, you can make the dough in a stand mixer or food processor.

7. Preheat the oven to 175°C.

8. Cut the dough into 6 pieces. On a well-floured work surface, roll each piece out to a ½ cm-thick circle. Slide your hands under the dough and gently loosen it. This encourages your dough to pre-shrink before you line your pie dish, so that it won't shrink in the oven. Roll out further if necessary, then line two 23 cm pie dishes with 2 dough circles and trim any excess pastry.

9. Fill each base with the cooled beef stew mixture. Do not exceed the height of the pastry. Cover the mixture with the remaining 2 dough circles and trim the edges. Use a fork to seal the base and the top together. Cut an X in the centre of each pie top so steam can be released. Brush the tops of the pies with a little beaten egg and a few sesame seeds, if using.

10. Bake for 30 minutes or until the pie tops are golden and the bottom is cooked through. Allow the pies to cool for at least 5–10 minutes before serving.

Serving Suggestion
Serve the pies with mashed potato, gravy and steamed greens.

Storage & Reheating
Allow to cool completely before chilling or freezing. The pies will keep for up to 1 week in the fridge or 2 months in the freezer.

Uncooked pies will keep for up to 3 months in the freezer or a day in the fridge. Allow the cooked pies to cool completely before chilling or freezing. They will keep for 1 week in the fridge or 2 months in the freezer.

The uncooked pies can be cooked from frozen. Preheat the oven to 180°C. Brush the top of the frozen pie with a little milk or lightly beaten egg and cook for around 40 minutes or until hot all the way through. Cover with foil if the pastry is browning too quickly.

If reheating a cooked pie from frozen, defrost overnight in the fridge. Preheat the oven to 180°C and cover the pie with foil. Bake until heated through evenly.

Pulled Pork

One pork shoulder makes enough for two or even three meals for a family of four, or a big pulled pork lunch for 6–8 people. The pulled pork takes 6 hours to cook but requires very little labour on your part (HOORAY!).

Ingredients

3 kg pork shoulder

1 tablespoon salt

1 teaspoon pepper

1 tablespoon smoked paprika

2 tablespoons brown sugar

Method

1. Preheat the oven to 150°C.
2. Place a piece of foil large enough to wrap your pork a couple of times on a work surface. Combine the salt, pepper, paprika and sugar in a small bowl. Rub the pork with the seasoning mix, then wrap tightly in the foil.
3. Place the pork in a large baking dish and cook for approximately 6 hours – the meat should pull away easily from the bone.
4. Shred the pork with two forks. It can then be cooled, portioned and frozen for future use.

Serving Suggestion

Serve pulled pork in soft white rolls with coleslaw.

Storage & Reheating

Allow to cool completely before chilling or freezing. The pork will keep for up to 1 week in the fridge or 2 months in the freezer.

To cook from frozen, defrost overnight in the fridge. Pan-fry the shredded meat in a splash of canola, sunflower or grapeseed oil until it takes on a gold hue and develops a crunchy, chewy texture.

Beef Noodle Stir-Fry

Ingredients

3 garlic cloves, finely chopped

2 tablespoons soy sauce

2 teaspoons sesame oil

2 teaspoons brown sugar

300 g beef bolar blade, trimmed and thinly sliced

2 x 500 g packs Hokkien-style yellow noodles

2 tablespoons canola, sunflower or grapeseed oil

1 bunch spring onions, tops cut into 4 cm-long pieces, ends discarded

1 red capsicum, julienned

2 carrots, julienned

3 tablespoons oyster sauce

Method

1. Combine the garlic with 1 tablespoon of the soy sauce, sesame oil and brown sugar in a large bowl. Add the beef and toss to coat in the marinade.

★ **At this point, the beef and the marinade can be transferred to a zip lock bag and frozen.**

2. Place the noodles in a large bowl or saucepan and pour over just-boiled water to cover. Gently loosen the noodles with two forks, then drain and set aside.

3. Heat the oil in a large heavy-based frying pan or wok over medium heat. Add the vegetables and stir-fry for a few minutes. Add the beef and stir-fry until cooked through.

4. Quickly add the noodles, oyster sauce and remaining soy sauce and stir through ingredients to combine. As soon as the noodles are coated, remove from the heat. Season to taste and serve.

Storage & Reheating

You should only freeze the uncooked marinated beef. Refrigerate for up to 5 days. For best results, keep the prepared vegetables in the fridge or prepare immediately prior to cooking. Unopened packets of noodles can be frozen for up to 1 month.

To cook from frozen, defrost the beef overnight in the fridge. Follow steps 3–4 to cook.

One-Tray Chicken Drumsticks

Ingredients

2 tablespoons olive oil, plus extra
   for greasing
3 garlic cloves, finely chopped
2 lemons, zested and thinly sliced
4 rosemary sprigs, leaves picked
2 tablespoons honey
1 teaspoon salt

½ teaspoon pepper
1 kg chicken drumsticks
6 large potatoes, each cut
   into 8–10 chunks
4 carrots, each cut into
   8–10 chunks

Method

1. Preheat the oven to 200°C. Grease a large heavy-based baking dish.
2. Combine 1 tablespoon of the olive oil with the garlic, lemon zest, rosemary, honey, salt and pepper in a large bowl. Add the chicken drumsticks and rub well to coat in the marinade.
3. Place the potatoes and carrots in the baking dish and drizzle over the remaining olive oil. Season with a little salt and pepper.
4. Lay the drumsticks over the top of the vegetables and top with the lemon slices.
5. Bake for 30–35 minutes or until the chicken is golden and cooked through.

Serving Suggestion

Serve with green salad leaves on the side.

Storage & Reheating

Allow to cool completely before chilling or freezing. This dish will keep for up to 5 days in the fridge or up to 1 month in the freezer.

If cooking from frozen, defrost overnight in the fridge. To reheat, cover with foil and place in a 200°C oven until evenly heated through.

Chicken Wing Soup

Make the chicken wing stock first so that the bones can be removed before adding the other soup ingredients. This will save you having to pick out any bones when you serve the soup.

Ingredients
Chicken wing stock
1 kg chicken wings
1 onion, chopped
2 garlic cloves, smashed

4 star anise
1 teaspoon salt

Soup
2 litres chicken wing stock
3 garlic cloves, smashed
4 cm piece ginger, thinly sliced,
1 bunch coriander, roots washed
and reserved, leaves roughly
chopped
3 spring onions, tops thinly sliced,
ends reserved

3 carrots, diced
4 celery stalks, diced
¾ cup rice – we prefer basmati but
you can use any variety
¼ white cabbage, shredded
soy sauce, to taste

Method
1. Place the chicken wings, onion, garlic and star anise in a large stockpot and pour over 3 litres water. Simmer over a low heat for at least 2 hours (removing any scum that rises to the surface with the back of a spoon) until the meat has fallen off the bones and the liquid is flavourful. Season with salt and black pepper, to taste.
2. Strain the stock into a large bowl. Set aside the chicken meat and discard the chicken bones.
3. Pour the chicken wing stock and 500 ml water into a clean stockpot and add the garlic, ginger, coriander roots and spring onion ends. Bring to a gentle simmer, add the carrot and celery and cook for about 10 minutes or until the vegetables are nearly soft.

4. Add the rice, cooked chicken and shredded cabbage and cook, stirring occasionally to prevent the rice from sticking, for about 10 minutes or until the rice is cooked through.
5. Season with soy sauce and black pepper, to taste. Finely grate a little fresh ginger over the top of the soup for an extra kick, if desired.
6. Scatter over the spring onion tops and coriander leaves and serve.

Storage & Reheating

Allow to cool completely before chilling or freezing. The soup will keep for 1 week in the fridge or up to 3 months in the freezer.

To cook from frozen, defrost overnight in the fridge. Reheat thoroughly in a microwave or saucepan.

Family Classics Menu

Family Classics Menu

Sometimes nothing else will do but a comforting Classic! Having these meals in the freezer are great for those nights when you just can't be bothered or you're too darned tired to cook but want something home-cooked and deeply comforting.

Meals

Rich Fish Pie

Goulash

Cottage Pie

Tuna Mornay Bake

Traditional Meatloaf

Sweet & Sour Meatballs

Apricot Chicken

Shopping List

Meat & Fish

600 g whiting fillet
600 g salmon fillet
1.5 kg chicken thighs, boneless
900 g pork mince
600 g beef skirt steak
1.5 kg beef mince

Fruit & Veg

6 onions
1 head garlic
12 large potatoes
7 carrots
3 red capsicums
1 bunch celery
1 bunch thyme
1 bunch rosemary
1 bunch dill

Dairy & Frozen

200 g plus 3 tablespoons butter
1.5 litres milk
700 g tasty cheese
2 eggs
1 cup frozen peas

Tins, Jars & Dry Goods

2 x 400 g tins diced tomatoes
3 cups jasmine rice
1 x 425 g tin tuna in oil or brine
1 x 400 ml tin apricot nectar
1 x 440 g tin pineapple rings or chunks in juice
2⅓ cups breadcrumbs
100 g dried apricots

Pantry Essentials

canola, sunflower or grapeseed oil
olive oil
850 ml beef stock
1 cup plain flour
1 tablespoon cornflour
3 tablespoons tomato paste
⅓ cup sugar
¼ cup white vinegar
salt
pepper
100 ml Worcestershire sauce
½ cup tomato sauce (ketchup)
¼ cup barbecue sauce
3 tablespoons soy sauce

Spices & Dried Herbs

2 tablespoons plus ½ teaspoon sweet paprika
pinch of curry powder
1 tablespoon dried oregano
½ teaspoon freshly ground nutmeg
2 bay leaves

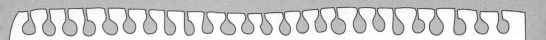

Serving Size
Each meal serves a family of 4 (approximately)

Preparation time
3 hours

Equipment
Preparation: sharp knives, chopping boards suitable for vegetables and fruit, meat and fish, kitchen scales, measuring cups and spoons, vegetable peeler, grater, mixing bowls in assorted sizes, rolling pin, whisk, mixing spoon.

Cooking: saucepans, frying pans, 2 large ceramic baking dishes, 2 small loaf tins or 1 large, heavy-based stockpot.

Storage: airtight containers suitable for freezing.

Storage & Reheating
All of these meals are freezer-friendly and will keep for up to 2 months in the freezer. Each meal should be defrosted the night before you plan to eat it, but don't panic if you forget and remember in the morning – just defrost them on the kitchen bench until dinnertime and then reheat fully. If you are sure you will eat all the dishes within the week, you can keep them all in the fridge.

Once-A-Week Cooking Preparation

	Total	Rich Fish Pie	Goulash	Cottage Pie
Fresh Produce				
Onions	6		1 thinly sliced	2 finely chopped
Garlic	1		2 cloves, thinly sliced	3 cloves, finely chopped
Potatoes	12	7 peeled and cut into 8 pieces each		5 peeled and cut into 4 pieces each
Carrots	7			3 finely diced
Capsicums	3		2 thinly sliced	
Celery	1		.	4 stalks, finely diced
Thyme	1			5 sprigs, leaves picked and finely chopped
Rosemary	1			
Dill	1	1 bunch, leaves finely chopped		
Cheese				
Tasty cheese	700 g	200 g, grated		200 g, grated
Meat & Fish				
Beef skirt steak	600 g		600 g, cut into 5–6 cm–long pieces	
Beef mince	1.5 kg			reserve 1 kg
Pork mince	900 g			
Chicken thighs	1.5 kg			

Tuna Mornay Bake	Traditional Meatloaf	Sweet & Sour Meatballs	Apricot Chicken
	1 finely chopped	1 finely chopped	1 finely chopped
	3 cloves, finely chopped		3 cloves, finely chopped
	2 grated	1 grated and 1 julienned	
		1 julienned	
		3 stalks, sliced	
3 sprigs, leaves picked	3 sprigs, leaves picked and finely chopped		4 sprigs, leaves picked and finely chopped
	3 sprigs, leaves picked and finely chopped		
200 g, grated	100 g, grated		
	reserve 500 g		
	reserve 400 g	reserve 500 g	
			1.5 kg, boneless, each thigh cut in half

Once-A-Week Cooking Plan

1. Preheat the oven to 200°C.

2. Place the whiting and salmon for the **Rich Fish Pie** in a greased ceramic baking dish and cover with 600 ml milk. Bake for 20–30 minutes or until the fish flakes easily. Reserve the milk.

3. Make the mashed potato toppings for the **Rich Fish Pie** and **Cottage Pie**.

4. Complete the **Rich Fish Pie** while the ingredients are still warm and bake for 30–40 minutes.

5. Next, prepare the **Goulash** as it has the longest cooking time. Brown the meat and prepare the sauce with the cooked vegetables. Slow-cook the dish 1½–2 hours.

6. Make the **Cottage Pie** and bake for 30–40 minutes.

7. Cook the rice for the **Tuna Mornay** and prepare the béchamel. Combine with the tinned tuna and grated cheese.

8. Prepare the **Traditional Meatloaf** mixture and bake for 35–40 minutes.

9. Make the meatballs for the **Sweet & Sour Meatballs**. Fry the meatballs and then prepare the sauce.

10. Finally, prepare the **Apricot Chicken**. Brown the meat and then prepare the sauce.

11. Allow all dishes to cool completely before chilling or freezing.

Rich Fish Pie

Ingredients

70 g butter, plus extra for greasing
600 g whiting fillet
600 g salmon fillet
600 ml milk
7 large potatoes, peeled and each
   cut into 8 pieces

1 teaspoon salt
2 tablespoons plain flour
1 bunch dill, leaves finely chopped
½ teaspoon freshly ground
   nutmeg
200 g tasty cheese, grated

Method

1. Preheat the oven to 200°C. Grease a large ceramic baking dish with butter.
2. Place the whiting and salmon in the dish and pour over the milk. Bake for 20–30 minutes or until the fish is cooked through.
3. Meanwhile, place the potatoes in a large stockpot and pour in enough water to cover. Add a pinch of salt and boil until tender. Drain and mash the potatoes with half of the butter and the salt.
4. When the fish is cooked, strain the milk and add one-quarter of it to the mash. Stir to combine. Flake the fish and leave in the baking dish.
5. Melt the remaining butter in the stockpot over medium heat until bubbling, then add the flour, stirring to combine. When the mixture resembles wet sand, add the remaining milk you used to cook the fish in. Stir the mixture constantly until it thickens, about 3–5 minutes from when it begins to bubble. Add the dill, grated nutmeg and stir to combine. Remove from the heat and season, to taste.
6. Pour the sauce over the flaked fish. Top pie with the mashed potato and sprinkle over the grated cheese.
7. Bake for 30–40 minutes or until bubbling and golden.

Serving Suggestion

Serve with baby peas.

Storage & Reheating

Allow to cool completely before chilling or freezing. The fish pie will keep for up to 1 week in the fridge or 1 month in the freezer.

If cooking from frozen, defrost overnight in the fridge. Cover with foil and place in a preheated 180°C oven until evenly heated through. Remove the foil for the last 10 minutes of cooking.

Goulash

Ingredients

50 g butter

1 tablespoon oil

600 g beef skirt steak, cut into
5–6 cm-long pieces

1 onion, thinly sliced

2 garlic cloves, thinly sliced

2 red capsicums, thinly sliced

2 tablespoons sweet paprika

1 bay leaf

2 tablespoons tomato paste

2 x 400 g tins diced tomatoes

150 ml beef stock

Method

1. Heat the butter and oil in a large heavy-based saucepan over medium–high heat. Add the beef and brown on all sides. Remove from the saucepan and set aside. If necessary, do this in batches to prevent the beef steaming instead of browning.
2. Add the onion and garlic to the pan and sauté until tender, about 5–7 minutes.
3. Return the beef to the pan, add the capsicum, paprika and bay leaf and stir for 1 minute. Add the tomato paste and stir through to combine. Allow to cook off for a couple of minutes, then add the tinned tomatoes and stock.
4. Bring the goulash to the boil, then lower the heat and simmer, covered, for 1½–2 hours, or until the beef is tender and the sauce has thickened.

Serving Suggestion

Serve the goulash over steamed rice, topped with sour cream and sprinkled with chopped parsley.

Storage & Reheating

Allow to cool completely before chilling or freezing. The goulash will keep for up to 1 week in the fridge or 2 months in the freezer.

To cook from frozen, defrost overnight in the fridge. Reheat gently and thoroughly in a microwave or saucepan.

Cottage Pie

Ingredients

3 tablespoons canola, sunflower or grapeseed oil

1 kg beef mince

2 onions, finely chopped

4 celery stalks, finely diced

3 carrots, finely diced

3 garlic cloves, finely chopped

4 tablespoons plain flour

1 tablespoon tomato paste

700 ml beef stock

80 ml Worcestershire sauce

5 thyme sprigs, leaves picked and finely chopped

1 bay leaf

5 large potatoes, peeled and each cut into 4 pieces

200 ml milk

3 tablespoons butter

200 g tasty cheese, grated

Method

1. Heat 1 tablespoon of the oil in a large heavy-based saucepan over medium heat. Add the mince and brown, using a wooden spoon to break up any lumps. Remove the mince from the pan and set aside.
2. Add the remaining oil along with the vegetables and garlic. Sauté for about 20 minutes or until soft. Add the flour and stir thoroughly to combine. Add the tomato paste, stir to combine and allow to cook off for 2 minutes.
3. Return the mince to the pan and pour over the beef stock. Increase the heat and bring to a simmer. Add the Worcestershire sauce, thyme leaves and bay leaf. Cook, uncovered, for 40–50 minutes or until the sauce has thickened and reduced. Season to taste and discard the bay leaf.
4. Preheat the oven to 200°C.
5. Meanwhile, place the potatoes in a large saucepan and cover with cold water. Bring to the boil over medium–high heat and cook until tender. Drain, allow to steam a little, then mash with the milk, butter and half of the cheese. Season, to taste.
6. Pour the meat mixture into a large ceramic or glass baking dish. Spread the mash over the top and sprinkle over the rest of the cheese.
7. Bake for 30–40 minutes or until the top is golden.

Serving Suggestion

Serve with steamed green vegetables or a salad.

Storage & Reheating

Allow to cool completely before chilling or freezing. The pie will keep for 1 week in the fridge or 2 months in the freezer.

If cooking from frozen, defrost overnight in the fridge. Preheat the oven to 180°C, cover the dish with foil and bake for 30 minutes. Remove the foil and bake for a further 10 minutes or until the top is crisp and golden.

Tuna Mornay

Ingredients

80 g butter, plus extra for greasing

3 cups jasmine rice

1 x 425 g tin tuna in oil or brine, drained

5 tablespoons plain flour

3 thyme sprigs, leaves picked

½ teaspoon sweet paprika

pinch of curry powder

½ teaspoon salt

½ teaspoon pepper

2½ cups milk

200 g tasty cheese, grated

1 cup breadcrumbs

Method

1. Preheat the oven to 200°C. Lightly butter a large casserole dish or ceramic baking dish.
2. Place the rice and 1.5 litres water in a medium-sized saucepan. Cover and bring to the boil over medium–high heat. Reduce the heat to low and cook, covered, for 18 minutes. Remove from the heat and set aside for 5 minutes before fluffing with a fork. Alternatively, cook the rice in a rice cooker.
3. Place half of the rice in the base of the casserole dish and top with half of the tuna.
4. Melt the butter in a small saucepan over medium–high heat until bubbling. Add the flour, thyme leaves, paprika, curry powder, salt and pepper and stir to combine. When the mixture resembles wet sand, whisk in the milk. Whisk the sauce constantly until it thickens, at least 3–5 minutes from the moment it starts to bubble. Remove from the heat and whisk in the cheese.
5. Pour half of the sauce over the tuna and rice in the casserole dish. Top with the remaining rice and tuna, then pour over the remaining cheese sauce.
6. Sprinkle over the breadcrumbs and bake for 30–40 minutes or until golden and bubbling on top.

Serving Suggestion

Serve with mashed potatoes and peas.

Storage & Reheating

Allow to cool completely before chilling or freezing. This dish will keep for 1 week in the fridge or 2 months in the freezer.

If cooking from frozen, defrost overnight in the fridge. Preheat the oven to 200°C, cover the dish with foil and bake until evenly heated through.

Traditional Meatloaf

Ingredients

500 g beef mince

400 g pork mince

1 onion, finely chopped

3 garlic cloves, finely chopped

2 carrots, grated

3 thyme sprigs, leaves picked and finely chopped

3 rosemary sprigs, leaves picked and finely chopped

1 egg

1 tablespoon Worcestershire sauce

1 cup breadcrumbs

1 teaspoon salt

1 teaspoon pepper

100 g tasty cheese, grated

½ cup tomato sauce (ketchup)

¼ cup barbecue sauce

Method

1. Preheat the oven to 200°C.
2. In a large bowl, combine all of the ingredients except the tomato sauce and barbecue sauce. Mix well with your hands to thoroughly combine. Press the mixture into two small loaf tins or one large loaf tin.
3. Combine the tomato sauce and barbecue sauce in a small bowl, then spread on top of the meatloaf.
4. Bake for 35–45 minutes, or until browned and caramelised on top and the meatloaf feels firm when pressed in the centre.

Serving Suggestion

Serve with mashed potatoes and gravy.

Storage & Reheating

Allow to cool completely before chilling or freezing. This dish will keep for up to 1 week in the fridge or 2 months in the freezer.

To cook from frozen, defrost overnight in the fridge. Preheat the oven to 180°C, cover the meatloaf with foil and bake for 30 minutes. Uncover and bake for a further 10 minutes or until the top is crisp.

Sweet & Sour Pork Meatballs

Ingredients

1 onion, finely chopped
2 carrots, 1 grated, 1 julienned,
500 g pork mince
1 egg
⅓ cup breadcrumbs
1 teaspoon salt
½ teaspoon pepper
3 tablespoons plain flour

3 tablespoons oil
1 red capsicum, julienned
3 celery stalks, finely sliced
1 x 440 g tin pineapple rings or
   chunks in juice
⅓ cup sugar
¼ cup white vinegar
1 tablespoon cornflour
3 tablespoons soy sauce

Method

1. Combine the onion, grated carrot and pork mince in a large bowl. Add the egg, breadcrumbs, salt and pepper and mix with your hands to combine.
2. Tip the flour onto a plate. Roll the meat mixture into palm-sized balls then roll in the flour.
3. Heat the oil in a large heavy-based saucepan over medium high heat. Add the meatballs and brown on all sides. Remove the meatballs from the heat and set aside.
4. Wipe the saucepan clean and return it to the heat. Add the julienned carrot, capsicum, celery and pineapple and one-quarter of the juice from the tin. Add the sugar, vinegar and ⅓ cup water. Bring to the boil then reduce to a simmer and cook for about 8 minutes or until the vegetables are tender.
5. In a small bowl, combine the cornflour and soy sauce to make a slurry. Add this to sauce and stir thoroughly to combine. The sauce will thicken after a few minutes.
6. Return the meatballs to the pan and simmer for 15–20 minutes or until cooked through.

Serving Suggestion

Serve with steamed jasmine rice on the side.

Storage & Reheating

Allow to cool completely before chilling or freezing. This dish will keep for up to 1 week in the fridge or 2 months in the freezer.

To cook from frozen, defrost overnight in the fridge. Preheat the oven to 180°C, cover the dish with foil and bake for 30 minutes until heated through.

Apricot Chicken

Ingredients

½ cup plain flour

1 teaspoon salt

½ teaspoon pepper

1.5 kg chicken thighs, boneless, cut in half

2 tablespoons olive oil

1 onion, finely chopped

3 garlic cloves, finely chopped

1 x 400 ml tin apricot nectar

4 thyme sprigs, leaves picked and finely chopped

100 g dried apricots, cut in half

1 tablespoon dried oregano

Method

1. Combine the flour, salt and pepper in a large bowl. Toss the chicken in the flour mixture and dust off any excess. Set aside.

2. Heat 1 tablespoon of the oil in a heavy-based saucepan or large frying pan with a lid over medium–high heat. Add the chicken and brown on all sides until golden. Remove the chicken from the pan and set aside.

3. Add the remaining oil to the pan and sauté the onion and garlic until softened. Add the apricot nectar and stir to combine. Bring the sauce to the boil and add the chicken. Reduce the heat to low and cook, covered, for 15 minutes.

4. Add the dried apricot, thyme and oregano and cook, uncovered, for a further 20 minutes or until the sauce has thickened. Season, to taste.

Serving Suggestion

Serve with couscous and salad.

Storage & Reheating

Allow to cool completely before chilling or freezing. The apricot chicken will keep for up to 1 week in the fridge or 2 months in the freezer.

If cooking from frozen, defrost overnight in the fridge. Preheat the oven to 180°C, cover the dish with foil and bake for 30 minutes until heated through.

7 Pies in 1 Day

━━ 7 Pies in 1 Day ━━

Pies and winter go hand-in-hand beautifully. You can prepare this plan and pop the pies in the freezer for the coming weeks. Pies make fabulous family dinners. Defrost, bake, and team up with some mash, gravy and lightly steamed greens and gather the family around.

MamaBaker Karen says:

> "I LOVE this plan! Having a pie stash in the freezer gives me an odd feeling of security. Put some lettuce on a plate, a couple of tomatoes, pull the warmed pie from the oven and boom! Dinner done. I tend to use one or two of the pies as weeknight dinners and one on the weekend for lunch, keeping the others for rainy days. We're a gluten-free family and I can easily substitute my favourite gluten-free pastry recipe, and any other filling or sauce ingredients containing gluten are simple to replace. The only recipe I can't adapt is the Spanakopita, but I make this anyway and share it with a friend."

This plan includes a great range of pies. Our recipes use a variety of pastries, including shortcrust, puff and filo, plus interesting topping combinations such as cornbread–mashed potato and scone–dumpling.

If you don't fancy making your own pastry, simply buy some store-bought shortcrust and puff. Filo is incredibly fiddly, so unless you've got stacks of time at your disposal, we recommend buying this from the shops!

Menu

Beef Pie

Chicken & Mushroom Pot Pie

Chicken Curry Pie

Vegetable & Bean Pie with Polenta Crust

Spanakopita

Individual Puffy Pork Pies

Tomato & Corn Pie

Shopping List

Meat & Fish	Fruit & Veg	Dairy & Frozen
800 g beef bolar blade 2.4 kg chicken breasts 600 g pork sausages	4 onions 2 heads garlic 3 large potatoes 9 carrots 2 parsnips 1 turnip or swede 3 corn cobs 1 bunch celery 32 button mushrooms 1 kg ripe tomatoes 1 bunch English spinach 4 spring onions 1 bunch basil 1 bunch dill 1 bunch chives 1 bunch rosemary 1 bunch thyme 1 bunch coriander 1 bunch parsley 1 lemon 1 apple	¾ milk 1.6 kg butter 100 ml cream ¾ cup plain yoghurt 12 eggs 200 g parmesan 300 g tasty cheese 300 g feta 150 g ricotta ⅓ cup mayonnaise 500 g puff pastry 1 cup frozen peas

Tins, Jars & Dry Goods	Pantry Essentials	Other Ingredients
1 x 450 ml tin coconut milk 2 x 400 g tins cannellini beans 2 x 400 g tins crushed tomatoes 100 g polenta 3 tbs breadcrumbs 1 tbs sesame seeds (optional)	canola, sunflower or grapeseed oil olive oil 2 cups beef stock 550 ml chicken stock 2 cups vegetable stock 1 jar tomato paste 2.2 kg flour 2 tsp cornflour 1 tsp baking powder salt pepper 1 tbs curry powder ¼ tsp ground nutmeg ½ tsp ground cumin 2 tbs tomato sauce (ketchup)	375 g filo pastry 1 cup white wine 1 cup red wine

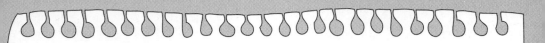

Serving Size
Each pie serves a family of 4 (approximately)

Preparation time
5 hours

Equipment
Preparation: sharp knives, chopping boards suitable for vegetables and fruit, meat and fish, kitchen scales, large 8-hole muffin tin, measuring cups and spoons, vegetable peeler, grater, sieve, large bowls, stand mixer (optional), food processor or blender, paper towel, whisk.
Cooking: 4 glass or ceramic baking dishes, 3 pie dishes, deep casserole dish, large deep baking dish, large heavy-based saucepans.
Storage: foil or plastic wrap.

Storage & Reheating
All of these pies are wonderfully freezer-friendly and will keep for 1–2 months in the freezer, depending on whether they are baked or unbaked. They just need to be defrosted the night before you plan to eat them. Don't panic if you forget to do this, just defrost the pie on the kitchen bench the day you intend to eat it, then reheat fully. Most of the pies will also last a few days or up to 1 week in the fridge. I like to keep pies for the first three nights of the week in the fridge and freeze the rest.

Once-A-Week Cooking Preparation

	Total	Beef Pie	Chicken & Mushroom Pot Pie	Chicken Curry Pie
Pastry				
Shortcrust pastry		combine and prepare the pastries		combine and prepare the pastries
Fresh Produce				
Onions	4	1 diced	1 finely chopped	1 chopped
Garlic	2	3 cloves, finely chopped	3 cloves, finely chopped	4 cloves, finely chopped
Potatoes	3			3 diced
Carrots	9	2 diced		2 diced
Parsnips	2			
Turnip or swede	1			
Corn	3			
Celery	1	4 stalks, diced		
Mushrooms	32	5 quartered	15 thinly sliced	
Tomatoes	1 kg			
English spinach	1			
Spring onions	4			
Basil	1			
Dill	1			
Chives	1			
Rosemary	1	4 sprigs, leaves picked and finely chopped		
Thyme	1		6 sprigs, leaves picked and finely chopped	
Coriander	1			1 bunch, stalks finely chopped, leaves roughly chopped
Parsley	½			
Apple	1			
Lemon	1			
Cheese				
Parmesan	200 g			
Tasty cheese	300 g			
Meat				
Pork sausages	600 g			
Chicken breasts	2.4 kg		1.8 kg, diced into 3 cm pieces	600 g, diced into 3 cm pieces
Beef bolar blade	800 g	800 g, trimmed and cut into 2 cm pieces		

Vegetable & Bean Pie with Polenta Crust	Spanakopita	Individual Puffy Pork Pies	Tomato & Corn Pie
			combine and prepare the pastries
1 finely chopped			
3 cloves, finely chopped			
3 finely diced		2 grated	
2 finely diced			
1 finely diced			
			3 cobs, kernels stripped
		3 stalks, finely diced	
12 sliced			
			1 kg, sliced 1 cm thick
	1 bunch, stems finely chopped, leaves roughly chopped		
	4, tops thinly sliced		
			1 bunch, leaves picked and roughly chopped
	1 bunch, leaves picked and finely chopped		
			1 bunch, finely chopped
4 sprigs, leaves picked and finely chopped			
4 sprigs, leaves picked and finely chopped			
		½ bunch, finely chopped	
		1 grated	
			1 juiced
100 g, grated	100 g, grated		
100 g grated			200 g, grated
		600 g, skins split and meat scooped out	

Once-A-Week Cooking Plan

1. Preheat the oven to 200°C. Place 4 large heavy-based saucepans on the stovetop.

2. Make the shortcrust pastry for the **Beef Pie**, **Chicken Curry Pie** and **Tomato & Corn Pie** and set aside in the fridge.

3. Prepare the **Beef Pie** filling first, as this takes the longest to cook. Simmer for 2 hours.

4. Make the fillings for the **Chicken & Mushroom Pot Pie** and **Chicken Curry Pie** and put them on to cook.

5. Next, make the filling for the **Vegetable & Bean Pie with Polenta Crust** and place on the heat.

6. Prepare the **Spanakopita** filling and fill the filo pastry. Once you have started the filo process it is best you complete the pie. Brush it with melted butter and set aside in the fridge. This prevents the filo drying out.

7. Set aside the fillings for the **Beef Pie**, **Chicken & Mushroom Pot Pie** and **Chicken Curry Pie** to cool completely.

8. Transfer the filling for the **Vegetable & Bean Pie with Polenta Crust** into a glass or ceramic baking dish and prepare the polenta topping. Pour the topping over the filling and bake in the oven.

9. Take the puff pastry sheets out of the freezer to defrost.

10. Roll out the pastry for the **Beef Pie, Chicken Curry Pie** and **Tomato & Corn Pie** and fill 3 pie dishes with the base pastry.

11. Prepare the filling for the **Individual Puffy Pork Pies** and cut out the pastry circles from the puff pastry. Assemble the pies and bake or freeze.

12. Prepare the **Tomato & Corn Pie** filling in one of the cases and then top with another layer of pastry and bake. Allow to cool completely before chilling or freezing.

13. Fill a baking dish with the **Chicken & Mushroom Pot Pie** filling and top with a couple of sheets of puff pastry. Bake or freeze.

14. Transfer the fillings for the **Chicken Curry Pie** and **Beef Pie** to separate pie dishes and top with more pastry. Bake or freeze.

15. Allow the cooked pies to cool completely before chilling or freezing.

Beef Pie

Ingredients

2 tablespoons canola, sunflower or grapeseed oil

800 g beef bolar blade, trimmed and cut in 2 cm pieces

1 onion, diced

2 carrots, diced

4 large celery stalks, diced

3 garlic cloves, finely chopped

3 tablespoons tomato paste

5 large button mushrooms, quartered

4 rosemary sprigs, leaves picked and finely chopped

1½ teaspoons salt

2 cups beef stock

black pepper

Shortcrust pastry

680 g plain flour

2 teaspoons salt

450 g cold butter, diced

225 ml very cold water

1 egg (optional)

sesame seeds (optional)

Method

1. To make the filling, heat the oil in a large heavy-based saucepan over medium heat. Add the beef and cook until browned. Remove the beef and set aside.

2. Return the pan to the heat. Add the onion, carrot, celery and garlic, and sauté until the onion is translucent.

3. Return the beef to the pan and add the tomato paste. Stir and allow to cook off for a few minutes. Add the mushrooms, rosemary and salt, then pour in the beef stock. Bring to a simmer and reduce to a low–medium heat for 2 hours, until the beef is very tender. Stir occasionally to ensure that the pie filling doesn't catch on the base of the pan. The sauce should be reduced to just cover the beef and vegetables.

4. Season the filling with salt and pepper, to taste. Transfer to a large dish and set aside to cool in the fridge.

5. Meanwhile, make the pastry. (You can use your own recipe, if you prefer.) Combine flour and salt in a large bowl. Using your hands, rub the butter into the flour until the mixture resembles coarse

breadcrumbs. Make a well in the mixture and add the cold water. Stir to combine and form into a smooth dough – it should not be wet or sloppy, so add a little more flour or water, if needed, to get the right consistency.

6. Transfer the dough to a lightly floured work surface and knead gently until a smooth dough is formed, being careful not to overwork it. (Alternatively, you can easily make the dough in a stand mixer or food processor.)

7. Wrap the dough in plastic wrap and set aside in the fridge for at least 1 hour. If you have prepared a bulk quantity of dough to use in the other recipes in this plan, then cut the dough into 6 pieces and set 4 pieces aside for the Chicken Curry Pie and the Tomato & Corn Pie. Otherwise, cut your dough in half.

8. Roll out the dough on a lightly floured work surface into 2 circles about ½ cm thick. Slide your hands under the dough and gently loosen it by moving your fingers. This allows your dough to pre-shrink before you line your pie dish, so that it won't shrink in the oven. Roll out further if necessary, then line your pie dish with the dough and trim any excess pastry.

9. Fill the dish with the cooled pie filling and top with the other pastry half. Trim any excess pastry and cut an X in the centre of the pie top to allow steam to escape. Brush the pastry with a little beaten egg and sprinkle with sesame seeds, if using.

★ **At this point, the pie can be frozen.**

10. Preheat the oven to 175°C.
11. Bake the pie for 30 minutes or until the top is golden and the bottom is cooked through. Allow your pie to cool for at least 5–10 minutes before serving.

Serving Suggestion
Serve with creamy mashed potatoes.

Storage & Reheating
Unbaked, the pie will keep for up to 5 days in the fridge or 2 months in the freezer. Allow the baked pie to cool completely before chilling

or freezing. It will keep for up to 1 week in the fridge or 2 months in the freezer.

To cook the unbaked pie from frozen, preheat the oven to 180°C. Brush the top of the pie with a little milk or lightly beaten egg and cook for about 40 minutes or until evenly heated through. Cover with foil if the pastry is browning too quickly.

To cook the baked pie from frozen, defrost overnight in the fridge. Preheat the oven to 180°C and cover the pie with foil. Bake until heated through evenly.

Chicken & Mushroom Pot Pie

Ingredients

1.8 kg chicken breasts, diced into 3 cm pieces

4 tablespoons plain flour

1 tablespoon olive oil

1 onion, finely chopped

3 garlic cloves, finely chopped

15 button mushrooms, thinly sliced

6 thyme sprigs, leaves picked and finely chopped

55 g butter, plus extra for greasing

1 cup white wine

300 ml chicken stock

100 ml cream

250 g puff pastry (2 sheets)

1 egg, beaten

Method

1. Preheat the oven to 200°C.
2. Place the chicken and flour in a large bowl and toss to combine.
3. Heat the oil in a large heavy-based saucepan over medium heat. Add the onion and garlic and cook, stirring frequently, until softened, about 7–8 minutes. Add the mushrooms and thyme and cook for 5 minutes. Add the chicken and stir to combine. Cook until the chicken is golden on all sides.
4. Push the mixture to one side and add the butter in the space left. Increase the heat and allow the butter to foam before stirring through the mixture. Add the wine and turn the heat up further to simmer for a couple of minutes. Add the chicken stock and cream and simmer 5–7 minutes, or until the mixture thickens. Season to taste.
5. Pour the mixture into a greased ceramic or glass pie dish.

★ **If you wish to freeze the pie unbaked, allow the mixture to cool completely before placing the puff pastry on top.**

6. Place the puff pastry sheets over the mixture and cut off any excess pastry. Brush the pastry with beaten egg and cut a small X in the centre of the pastry to release steam.
7. Bake for 20–30 minutes or until the pastry is puffed up and golden.

Serving Suggestion

Serve with creamy mashed potatoes and steamed vegetables.

Storage & Reheating

Unbaked, the pie will keep for up to 5 days in the fridge or 2 months in the freezer. Allow the cooked pie to cool completely before chilling or freezing. It will keep for up to 1 week in the fridge or 1 month in the freezer.

To cook the unbaked pie from frozen, preheat the oven to 180°C. Brush the top of the pie with a little milk or lightly beaten egg and cook for about 40 minutes or until evenly heated through. Cover with foil if the pastry is browning too quickly.

To cook the baked pie from frozen, defrost overnight in the fridge. Preheat the oven to 180°C and cover the pie with foil. Bake until heated evenly through.

Chicken Curry Pie

Ingredients

3 tablespoons butter

600 g chicken breasts, diced into 3 cm pieces

1 onion, chopped

2 carrots, diced

1 bunch coriander, stalks finely chopped, leaves roughly chopped

4 garlic cloves, finely chopped

3 tablespoons tomato paste

1 tablespoon curry powder

2 tablespoons flour

1 x 450 ml tin coconut milk

1 cup chicken stock

3 large potatoes, diced

1 cup frozen peas

Shortcrust pastry

680 g plain flour

2 teaspoons salt

450 g cold butter, diced

225 ml very cold water

1 egg (optional)

sesame seeds (optional)

Method

1. Melt 1 tablespoon of the butter in a large heavy-based saucepan over medium heat. Add the chicken to the pan in batches and cook, stirring frequently, until browned. Remove from the pan and set aside.

2. Add the onion, carrot and coriander stalks to the pan and cook until the onion is translucent. Add the garlic and the tomato paste and allow to cook off for 2 minutes. Stir through the curry powder and flour and cook for a further 3–4 minutes. Add the coconut milk and chicken stock and cook, stirring constantly, for about 8 minutes until the sauce has thickened.

3. Return the chicken to the pan, add the potato and cook for a further 5 minutes. Add the peas and the coriander leaves and season, to taste. Transfer the filling to a heatproof dish and set aside in the fridge to cool.

4. Meanwhile, make the pastry. (You can use your own recipe, if you prefer.) Combine flour and salt in a large bowl. Using your hands, rub the butter into the flour until the mixture resembles coarse breadcrumbs. Make a well in the mixture and add the cold water.

Stir to combine and form into a smooth dough – it should not be wet or sloppy, so add a little more flour or water, if needed, to get the right consistency.

5. Transfer the dough to a lightly floured work surface and knead gently until a smooth dough is formed, being careful not to overwork it. (Alternatively, you can easily make this dough in a stand mixer or food processor.)

6. Wrap the dough in plastic wrap and set aside in the fridge for at least 1 hour. If you have prepared a bulk quantity of dough to use in the other recipes in this plan, then cut the dough into 6 pieces and set 4 pieces aside for the Beef Pie and the Tomato & Corn Pie. Otherwise, cut your dough in half.

7. Roll out the dough on a lightly floured work surface into 2 circles about ½ cm thick. Slide your hands under the dough and gently loosen it by moving your fingers. This allows your dough to pre-shrink before you line your pie dish, so that it won't shrink in the oven. Roll out further if necessary, then line your pie dish with the dough and trim any excess pastry.

8. Fill the pie dish with the cooled pie filling and top with the other pastry half. Trim any excess pastry and cut an X in the centre of the pie top to allow steam to escape.

★   **At this point, the unbaked pie can be frozen.**

9. Preheat the oven to 175°C.

10. Bake for 30 minutes or until the pie top is golden and the bottom is cooked through. Allow the pie to cool for at least 5–10 minutes before serving.

Serving Suggestion

Serve with wilted greens sautéed in chilli, garlic and ginger.

Storage & Reheating

Unbaked, the pie will keep for up to 5 days in the fridge or 2 months in the freezer. Allow the baked pie to cool completely before chilling or freezing. It will keep for up to 1 week in the fridge or 1 month in the freezer.

To cook the unbaked pie from frozen, preheat the oven to 180°C. Brush the top of the pie with a little milk or lightly beaten egg and cook for about 40 minutes or until evenly heated through. Cover with foil if the pastry is browning too quickly.

To cook the baked pie from frozen, defrost overnight in the fridge Preheat the oven to 180°C and cover the pie with foil. Bake until heated evenly through.

Vegetable & Bean Pie with Polenta Crust

Ingredients

2 tablespoons olive oil

1 onion, finely chopped

3 garlic cloves, finely chopped

3 carrots, finely diced

2 parsnips, finely diced

1 turnip or swede, finely diced

12 button mushrooms, sliced

4 rosemary sprigs, leaves picked and finely chopped

4 thyme sprigs, leaves picked and finely chopped

3 tablespoons tomato paste

1 cup red wine

2 x 400 g tins cannellini beans, drained

2 cups vegetable stock

2 x 400 g cans crushed tomatoes

2 teaspoons cornflour mixed with 2 teaspoons water

Polenta Crust

2 eggs

¾ cup plain yoghurt

100 g tasty cheese, grated

100 g plain flour

1 teaspoon baking powder

100 g polenta

100 g parmesan, grated

Method

1. Heat the olive oil in a large heavy-based saucepan over medium heat. Add the onion and garlic and sauté for 5 minutes until the onion is translucent. Add the vegetables and herbs and cook for 15 minutes, stirring occasionally, until tender. Add the tomato paste and allow to cook off for 2 minutes. Add the wine and increase the heat to high. Simmer for 5 minutes. Add the drained beans, stock, crushed tomatoes and cornflour mixture.

2. Bring to the boil and simmer for 20 minutes or until the sauce is thick and slightly reduced. Season, to taste. Pour the mixture into a glass or ceramic baking dish.

3. Preheat the oven to 200°C.

4. To make the polenta crust, whisk the eggs and yoghurt in a large bowl. Add the tasty cheese, flour, baking powder and polenta. Season with a little salt and pepper.
5. Spread the topping over the pie filling and sprinkle with the parmesan.
6. Bake for 20–30 minutes or until the top is golden and the edges are bubbling.

Serving Suggestion
Serve with a fresh green salad.

Storage & Reheating
For best results freeze or refrigerate once cooked. Allow to cool completely before chilling or freezing. The pie will keep for up to 1 week in the fridge or 2 months in the freezer.

To cook from frozen, preheat the oven to 180°C. Cover the pie with foil and bake for 30 minutes or until evenly heated through.

Spanakopita

This is a much-loved Greek classic: a rich filling of spinach and cheese, spiked with fragrant dill, layered between sheets of filo pastry.

Ingredients

300 g feta

150 g ricotta

1 bunch dill, leaves picked and finely chopped

4 spring onions, tops thinly sliced

5 eggs, beaten

3 tablespoons dry breadcrumbs

1 teaspoon salt

½ teaspoon black pepper

1 bunch English spinach, stalks finely chopped, leaves roughly chopped

125 g melted butter

100 g parmesan, grated

375 g pack fresh filo pastry

¼ cup olive oil

Method

1. Preheat the oven to 180°C. Lightly grease a large 20 cm x 30 cm baking dish with some of the melted butter.
2. In a large bowl, combine the feta, ricotta, dill, spring onion, eggs, breadcrumbs, salt and pepper and olive oil. Mix well with your hands. Add the chopped spinach leaves and stems and mix to combine.
3. Lay out the filo sheets and keep under a tea towel to prevent them drying out as you make the spanakopita.
4. Line the baking dish with sheets of filo so that they cover the base and overhang the edges. Brush with a little melted butter, then continue with more filo sheets and butter until you have used half the pastry.
5. Press the spinach and cheese mixture gently into the pastry base. Top with more filo and butter layers. Butter the top pastry sheet generously with butter.
6. Using a sharp knife, score the pastry in a diamond pattern, or square if you prefer. This makes cutting and serving the fragile pastry much easier.

★   **At this point, the spanakopita can be frozen.**

7. Bake for 45–60 minutes or until the top is golden. Cover the dish with foil if it is browning too quickly.

Storage & Reheating

Unbaked, the spanakopita will keep for up to 1 week in the fridge or 2 months in the freezer. Allow the baked pie to cool completely before chilling or freezing. It will keep for up to 1 week in the fridge or 2 months in the freezer.

To cook the unbaked pie from frozen, preheat the oven to 180°C. Brush the top of the pie with a little milk or lightly beaten egg and cook for about 40 minutes or until evenly heated through. Cover with foil if the pastry is browning too quickly.

To cook the baked pie from frozen, defrost overnight in the fridge. Preheat the oven to 180°C and cover the pie with foil. Bake until evenly heated through.

Individual Puffy Pork Pies

Ingredients

olive oil, for greasing

600 g pork sausages, skins split and meat scooped out

3 celery stalks, finely diced

2 carrots, grated

1 apple, grated

½ bunch parsley, leaves picked and finely chopped

¼ teaspoon ground nutmeg

½ teaspoon ground cumin

2 tablespoons tomato sauce (ketchup)

½ teaspoon pepper

1 teaspoon salt

250 g frozen puff pastry sheets

1 egg, beaten

Method

1. Preheat the oven to 200°C. Grease a large 8-hole muffin tin.
2. Combine the sausage meat, celery, carrot, parsley, nutmeg, cumin tomato sauce and salt and pepper in a large bowl.
3. Using a biscuit cutter, cut 8 circles of puff pastry large enough to completely line the inside of the muffin holes with some overhang. Gently press the pastry into the holes and spoon the meat mixture on top, distributing evenly.
4. Cut another 8 puff pastry circles to make pastry lids, then cut an X in the centre of each circle. Brush the edge of the pastry base with beaten egg before pressing on the lids. Press the edges together with the back of a fork to make a decorative and well-sealed crust. Brush the tops with more beaten egg.

* **At this point, the pies can be frozen.**

5. Bake for 30–40 minutes or until the tops are golden brown.

Serving Suggestion

Serve with a side of chutney and some crunchy lettuce leaves.

Storage & Reheating

Unbaked, the frozen pies will keep for up to 2 months in the freezer and 5 days in the fridge.

Allow the baked pies to cool completely before chilling or baking. They will keep for up to 1 week in the fridge or 2 months in the freezer.

Unbaked frozen pies should be defrosted for at least 4–6 hours before baking. Preheat the oven to 200°C and bake for 30–40 minutes or until the tops are golden.

To cook baked pies from frozen, defrost for at least 6 hours. Preheat the oven to 200°C and bake for 20 minutes.

Tomato & Corn Pie

Ingredients

1 kg ripe tomatoes, sliced 1 cm thick

1 teaspoon salt

juice of 1 lemon

⅓ cup mayonnaise

3 corn cobs, kernels stripped and roughly chopped

1 bunch basil, leaves roughly chopped

1 bunch chives, finely chopped

1 tablespoon butter, melted

¾ cup milk

200 g tasty cheese, grated

½ teaspoon black pepper

Shortcrust pastry

680 g plain flour

2 teaspoons salt

450 g cold butter, diced

225 ml very cold water

1 egg (optional)

sesame seeds (optional)

Method

1. Grease a glass or ceramic pie dish.
2. Place the tomato on paper towels and sprinkle lightly with a little salt. Set aside.
3. Whisk the lemon juice and mayonnaise in a large bowl and set aside.
4. To make the pastry (you can use your own recipe, if you prefer), combine the flour and salt in a large bowl. Using your hands, rub the butter into the flour until the mixture resembles coarse breadcrumbs. Make a well in the mixture and add the cold water. Stir to combine and form into a smooth dough – it should not be wet or sloppy, so add a little more flour or water, if needed, to get the right consistency.
5. Transfer the dough to a lightly floured work surface and knead gently until a smooth dough is formed, being careful not to overwork it. (Alternatively, you can easily make this dough in a stand mixer or food processor.)
6. Wrap the dough in plastic wrap and set aside in the fridge for at least 1 hour. If you have prepared a bulk quantity of dough to use in the other recipes in this plan, then cut the dough into 6 pieces and set 4 pieces aside for the Beef Pie and the Chicken Curry Pie. Otherwise, cut your dough in half.

7. Roll out the dough on a lightly floured work surface into 2 circles about ½ cm thick. Slide your hands under the dough and gently loosen it by moving your fingers. This allows your dough to pre-shrink before you line your pie dish, so that it won't shrink in the oven. Roll out further if necessary, then line your pie dish with the dough and trim any excess pastry.

8. Layer half of the tomatoes in the pie, then top with half of the corn, half the basil and chives and a little salt and pepper. Repeat with the remaining ingredients. Sprinkle over half the cheese, and then top with the mayonnaise mixture. Sprinkle over the remaining cheese.

9. Top the pie with the other pastry circle. Trim and press the edges together to seal. Cut an X in the centre of the pie top to allow steam to escape. Brush the pastry with a little beaten egg and sprinkle over some sesame seeds, if using

★ **At this point, the pie can be frozen.**

10. Preheat the oven to 180°C.

11. Bake for 30–40 minutes or until the crust is golden. Allow to cool before serving.

Serving Suggestion

Serve with buttered steamed vegetables.

Storage & Reheating

The unbaked or baked pie will keep for up to 5 days in the fridge or 1 month in the freezer. Allow to cool completely before chilling or freezing.

To cook the unbaked pie from frozen, preheat the oven to 180°C. Brush the top of the pie with a little milk or lightly beaten egg and cook for about 40 minutes or until evenly heated through. Cover with foil if the pastry is browning too quickly.

To cook the baked pie from frozen, defrost overnight in the fridge. Preheat the oven to 180°C and cover the pie with foil. Bake until evenly heated through.

Cooked Breakfasts

Cooked Breakfasts

Mornings can be absolutely crazy and even more so if you are sleep-deprived and have school-aged kids who need packing off to school. Ideally, we would all love our kids to start their day with a belly full of warm, nourishing brekkie to sustain them throughout the day. And for us too! Sometimes it's just not possible to manage but this plan can help you make yummy warm breakfasts ahead of time and bring some peace back to the start of the day.

Menu

Breakfast Bagel Buns

Breakfast Pizzas

Savoury Bread Pudding

Breakfast Fruit Crumble

Cheesy Sausage, Rice & Zucchini Gratin

Home Fries & Eggs

Short-Cut 'Baked' Beans

Shopping List

Meat & Fish	Fruit & Veg	Dairy & Frozen
4 chorizo sausages 14 rashers bacon 100 g smoked salmon 100 g shaved ham	3 onions 1 head garlic 1 kg red or blue potatoes 3 zucchinis 1 red capsicum 1 green capsicum 12 large mushrooms 3 handfuls baby spinach 2 spring onions 1 bunch chives 1 bunch dill 1 bunch rosemary 7 large apples	50 g parmesan 300 g mozzarella 200 g Swiss cheese 250 g cream cheese 625 ml milk 17 eggs 150 g butter

Tins, Jars & Dry Goods	Pantry Essentials	Other Ingredients
2 x 400 g tins crushed tomatoes 4 x 400 g tins cannellini beans 1 cup rolled oats 1 cup desiccated or flaked coconut ½ cup jasmine rice 2 tbs sesame seeds	canola, sunflower or grapeseed oil olive oil 1.35 kg flour 4 tsp dry active yeast 120 g tomato paste ¼ cup caster sugar ½ cup brown sugar salt pepper 2 tbs mustard 2 tbs maple syrup 2 tbs Worcestershire sauce ½ tsp sweet paprika ½ nutmeg 1 tbs plus 1 tsp ground cinnamon	loaf stale bread

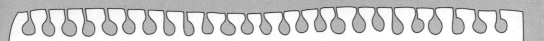

Serving Size
Each meal serves a family of 4 (approximately)

Preparation time
3 hours

Equipment
Preparation: sharp knives, chopping boards, kitchen scales, measuring cups and spoons, vegetable peeler, grater, mixing bowls in assorted sizes, rolling pin, whisk, mixing spoon, colander, pastry brush.
Cooking: saucepans, 4 ceramic casserole or baking dishes, baking trays, pizza trays (optional).
Storage: airtight containers suitable for freezing or zip lock bag/s.

Storage & Reheating
Most of the dishes in this plan will keep for several days to 1 week in the fridge. If you plan to eat the meals within the week, there is no need to freeze them.

All of these meals are also freezer-friendly and can be stored for 1–2 months in the freezer. Some need to be defrosted overnight or on the morning you plan to eat them, while other items can be baked from frozen.

Once-A-Week Cooking Preparation

	Total	Breakfast Bagel Buns	Breakfast Pizzas	Savoury Bread Pudding
Doughs				
Bagel and pizzas doughs		combine and prepare the doughs, and set aside to rise for 1–2 hours		
Fresh Produce				
Onions	3			
Garlic	1			
Potatoes	1 kg			
Zucchinis	3			
Red capsicum	1			
Green capsicum	1			
Mushrooms	12		12 thickly sliced	
Spring onions	2			
Chives	1	½ bunch, finely chopped		½ bunch, finely chopped
Dill	1	1 bunch, finely chopped		
Rosemary	1			
Apples	7			
Cheese				
Parmesan	50 g			
Mozzarella	300 g		200 g, grated	
Swiss cheese	200 g			200 g, grated
Meat & Fish				
Chorizo sausages	4		2 peeled and thickly sliced	
Bacon	14		8 rashers, roughly chopped	
Smoked salmon	100 g	100 g, roughly diced		
Shaved ham	100 g	100g, roughly diced		

Breakfast Fruit Crumble	Cheesy Sausage, Rice & Zucchini Gratin	Home Fries & Eggs	Short-Cut 'Baked' Beans
	1 finely chopped	1 roughly chopped	1 finely chopped
	3 cloves, finely chopped		3 cloves, finely chopped
		1 kg, cut into 2-cm chunks	
	3 grated		
		1 diced	
		1 diced	
		2 thinly sliced	
		3 sprigs, leaves picked and roughly chopped	
7 peeled, cored and cut into 2–3 cm chunks			
	50 g, grated		
	100 g, grated		
	2 peeled and thinly sliced		
			6 rashers, thinly sliced

Once-A-Week Cooking Plan

1. Combine and prepare the doughs for the **Breakfast Bagel Buns** and **Breakfast Pizzas**. Set aside to rise for 1–2 hours.

2. Preheat the oven to 200°C. Grease 4 ceramic casserole dishes.

3. Make the filling for the **Breakfast Bagel Buns** and place in the freezer.

4. Prepare the **Savoury Bread Pudding** egg mixture and soak the bread.

5. Cook the apples for the **Breakfast Fruit Crumble**. Set aside to cool.

6. Make the **Cheesy Sausage**, **Rice & Zucchini Gratin** and bake for 30 minutes.

7. Prepare the **Home Fries & Eggs** and bake alongside the gratin.

8. Make the **Short-Cut 'Baked' Beans**.

9. Reduce the oven temperature to 180°C.

10. Finish the **Savoury Bread Pudding** and place in the oven to bake.

11. Once the dough is ready, make the **Breakfast Pizzas**.

12. Roll out the dough for the **Breakfast Bagel Buns** and fill with the frozen cream cheese and salmon or ham balls.

13. Allow all dishes to cool completely before chilling or freezing.

Breakfast Bagel Buns

Ingredients
Dough
550 g plain flour, plus extra for kneading and dusting

2 teaspoons salt

2 tablespoons olive oil

2 teaspoons dry active yeast

370 ml warm water

Filling
250 g cream cheese, at room temperature

1 bunch dill, finely chopped

½ bunch chives, finely chopped

1 teaspoon salt

100 g smoked salmon, roughly diced

100 g shaved ham, roughly diced

Topping
1 egg, beaten

2 tablespoons sesame seeds

Method
1. To make the dough, place the flour, salt and olive oil in the bowl of a stand mixer or large bowl.
2. In a separate jug or bowl, add the yeast to the warm water and set aside for 10 minutes until the mixture begins to froth. Pour into the flour and mix until a rough dough forms. If you are using a stand mixer, knead the dough for 5 minutes. Alternatively, if you are making the dough by hand, scrape the dough onto a well-floured surface and knead for about 8–10 minutes.
3. Scrape the dough into a large lightly oiled bowl and cover with plastic wrap. Set aside for 1–2 hours or until doubled in size.
4. To make the fillings, combine the cream cheese, dill, chives and salt in a large bowl. Place the smoked salmon in separate bowls and add half of the cream cheese mixture to each bowl. Mix well and season further to taste.
5. Roll each mixture into 8 balls and place on a baking tray lined with baking paper. Place the tray in the freezer until the fillings are frozen.

6. Punch down the dough and divide into 16 equal pieces. On a well-floured surface, roll each piece into a ball and then flatten with a rolling pin to about 1 cm thick.
7. Place a frozen ball of filling in the centre of each dough round. Pull the dough up around the filling and press the edges together to seal tightly.

★ **At this point, the bagel buns can be frozen. Transfer to a baking tray and set aside in the freezer. Once frozen, pop them in a zip lock bag and return to the freezer. Unbaked bagels should be frozen if not baking immediately as they will continue to rise.**

8. Preheat the oven to 180°C. Line a baking tray with baking paper.
9. Place the bagels seam side down and at least 4 cm apart on the baking tray. Brush with beaten egg and sprinkle with sesame seeds.
10. Bake for 15–20 minutes or until puffed up and golden brown (the cheese will inevitably ooze a little).

Storage & Reheating

Baked bagels can be stored for up to 2 months in the freezer and up to 3 days in the fridge

Partially defrost the bagels before baking. Preheat oven to 200°C, place bagels in a baking tray, cover with foil and bake until thoroughly heated through.

Breakfast Pizzas

Ingredients
Dough

550 g plain flour, plus extra for kneading and dusting

2 teaspoons salt

2 teaspoons dry active yeast

2 tablespoons olive oil

370 ml warm water

Topping

100 g tomato paste

1 tablespoon brown sugar

1 teaspoon salt

8 bacon rashers, roughly chopped

2 chorizo sausages, peeled and thickly sliced

12 large mushrooms, thickly sliced

200 g mozzarella, grated

3 handfuls baby spinach

6 eggs

Method

1. To make the dough, place the flour, salt and olive oil in the bowl of a stand mixer or large bowl.
2. In a separate jug or bowl, add the yeast to the warm water and set aside for 10 minutes until the mixture begins to froth. Pour into the flour and mix until a rough dough forms. If you are using a stand mixer, knead the dough for 5 minutes. Alternatively, if you are making the dough by hand, scrape the dough onto a well-floured surface and knead for about 8–10 minutes.
3. Scrape the dough into a large lightly oiled bowl and cover with plastic wrap. Set aside for 1–2 hours or until doubled in size.
4. Combine the tomato paste, sugar, salt and 4 tablespoons water in a small bowl.
5. Preheat the oven to 200°C.
6. Divide the dough into 2 pieces and roll each piece out to a 1½–2 cm-thick circle. Lay each pizza base on a baking tray or pizza tray lightly dusted with flour.
7. Spread each base with a light coating of the tomato sauce. Form the bacon into a square around the edge of the pizza bases. Scatter

over the sliced chorizo, mushroom, grated cheese and baby spinach (but if you plan to freeze the pizzas, omit the spinach at this step). Carefully form three indents in the filling on each base.

* **You can freeze the pizzas at this point.**

8. Place the spinach (if not already used) and crack an egg into each indent (the filling around it should help the egg from running everywhere).
9. Bake for 15–20 minutes or until the cheese is crisp and melted and the eggs are set.

Storage & Reheating

Allow to cool completely before chilling or freezing. The pizzas will keep for up to 1 week in the fridge or 1 month in the freezer. If freezing unbaked, freeze from step 7 after making indents in base. Omit spinach and eggs until time of cooking. To bake from frozen, add the eggs and spinach to the indents. Reheat thoroughly in a 200°C oven, adding more cheese if necessary until the eggs are set and the cheese is bubbling and golden brown.

Savoury Bread Pudding

Ingredients

butter, for greasing
6 eggs
500 ml milk
2 tablespoons Dijon mustard
1 teaspoon salt
½ teaspoon pepper

½ bunch chives, finely chopped
1 medium-sized loaf stale bread, sliced
200 g Swiss cheese, grated
½ nutmeg, freshly grated

Method

1. Grease a ceramic baking dish with butter.
2. In a large bowl, whisk the eggs, milk and mustard. Season with half of the salt and half of the pepper. Stir in the chives.
3. Arrange half of the bread slices, overlapping, in the dish. Pour over half of the egg mixture and sprinkle over half of the cheese. Place the remaining bread slices on top, then add the rest of the milk mixture and cheese. Press gently to help the bread soak up the liquid. Set aside to soak for 30–60 minutes.
4. Preheat the oven to 180°C.
5. Bake the bread pudding for 45–60 minutes, or until it is puffed up and golden brown.

Storage & Reheating

Allow to cool completely before chilling or freezing. This dish will keep for up to 1 week in the fridge or 1 month in the freezer. You can also put the unbaked bread pudding in the fridge overnight and bake it the next morning.

There is no need to defrost this dish. Place in the oven and turn the temperature to 180°C. Heat until evenly warmed through and golden brown on top.

Breakfast Fruit Crumble

Ingredients

Filling

7 large apples, peeled, cored and cut into 2–3 cm chunks

¼ cup caster sugar

1 teaspoon ground cinnamon

Topping

1 cup plain flour

½ cup brown sugar

1 cup rolled oats

1 cup desiccated or flaked coconut

1 tablespoon ground cinnamon

½ teaspoon salt

120 g butter, plus extra for greasing

Method

1. Preheat the oven to 180°C. Grease a ceramic or glass baking dish.
2. To make the filling, tip the apples into a large saucepan and toss with the sugar and cinnamon. Cook over medium heat until the apples are just tender, about 10 minutes. Remove from the heat and set aside to cool.
3. To make the topping, combine the flour, sugar, oats, coconut, cinnamon and salt in a large bowl. Rub the butter into the dry mixture until it resembles large breadcrumbs.
4. Arrange the apple mixture in the baking dish and spread the crumble mixture over the top.
5. Bake for 25–35 minutes or until the topping is brown and crisp.

Serving Suggestion

Serve the crumble with a dollop of honey-sweetened Greek yoghurt.

Storage & Reheating

Allow to cool completely before chilling or freezing. The crumble will keep for up to 10 days in the fridge or 2 months in the freezer.

There is no need to defrost this dish. Place in the oven and turn the temperature to 180°C. Heat until evenly warmed through and golden brown on top.

Cheesy Sausage, Rice & Zucchini Gratin

Ingredients

3 zucchinis, grated

2 teaspoons salt

5 tablespoons olive oil

2 chorizo sausages, peeled and
    thinly sliced

1 onion, finely chopped

3 garlic cloves, finely chopped

3 tablespoons flour

½ cup jasmine rice

50 g parmesan, grated

100 g mozzarella, grated

½ cup milk

Method

1. Place the grated zucchini in a colander and toss through the salt. Set
    the colander over a bowl and set aside for 15–20 minutes (this helps
    to draw moisture from the zucchini). Squeeze out and reserve as
    much liquid as possible from the zucchini, then transfer the zucchini
    to a bowl. Keep the liquid and set aside.

2. Heat 2 tablespoons of the olive oil in a large saucepan over medium
    heat. Add the chorizo, onion and garlic and sauté for 5 minutes, or
    until the sausage starts to crisp and the onion is translucent. Add the
    zucchini and cook for 7 minutes, until tender. Add the flour and stir
    for 3 minutes. Remove from the heat and set aside.

3. Half-fill a small saucepan with water and add the rice. Boil for
    5 minutes, then drain and set aside.

4. Preheat the oven to 200°C.

5. Return the saucepan with the zucchini mixture to a medium heat.
    Add zucchini liquid to the pan. Bring to a simmer and stir. Add the
    rice and parmesan and stir to combine. Season, to taste.

6. Generously oil a ceramic or glass baking dish with the remaining
    olive oil. Pour the mixture into the dish and sprinkle over the
    mozzarella.

7. Bake for 30 minutes or until the top is golden and bubbling. When
    done, the rice should have absorbed the liquid and the gratin should
    have a thick texture.

Storage & Reheating

Allow to cool completely before chilling or freezing. The gratin will keep for up to 1 week in the fridge or 1 month in the freezer.

If cooking from frozen, defrost overnight in the fridge. To reheat, sprinkle 4 tablespoons of water or milk over the gratin and bake at 170°C for 15–20 minutes until thoroughly heated through.

Home Fries & Eggs

Ingredients

3 tablespoons olive oil, for greasing

1 kg red or blue potatoes, cut into 2–3 cm chunks

1 onion, roughly chopped

1 red capsicum, diced

1 green capsicum, diced

2 spring onions, thinly sliced, plus extra to garnish, if desired

3 rosemary sprigs, leaves picked and roughly chopped

½ teaspoon sweet paprika

1 teaspoon salt

½ teaspoon pepper

4 eggs

Method

1. Preheat the oven to 200°C. Grease a large heavy-based baking dish with 2 tablespoons of the olive oil.

2. Toss in the potato, onion, capsicum and rosemary. Season with the sweet paprika, salt and pepper, and toss with your hands to coat and combine.

3. Bake for 1 hour or until the potato is golden and crisp.

★ **Once completely cool, you can refrigerate or freeze the home fries at this point.**

4. Fry the eggs in the remaining olive oil and serve with a portion of home fries. Garnish with extra spring onion, if desired.

Storage & Reheating

Allow the home fries to cool completely before chilling or freezing. They will keep for up to 1 week in the fridge or 1 month in the freezer.

There is no need to defrost this dish. Place in the oven and turn the temperature to 200°C. Heat until evenly warmed through.

Short-Cut 'Baked' Beans

Ingredients

2 tablespoons oil

6 bacon rashers, thinly sliced

1 onion, finely chopped

3 garlic cloves, finely chopped

1 tablespoon tomato paste

2 tablespoons Worcestershire sauce

2 tablespoons maple syrup

2 x 400 g tins crushed tomatoes

4 x 400 g tins cannellini beans, drained

1 teaspoon salt

½ teaspoon pepper

Method

1. Heat the oil in a large heavy-based saucepan over medium heat.
2. Add the bacon, onion, garlic and cook, stirring frequently, until the onion is translucent and the bacon crisp. Add the remaining ingredients and stir well to combine.
3. Simmer for 15 minutes until sauce is thick and fragrant.

Serving Suggestion

Serve the beans with hot buttered toast.

Storage & Reheating

Allow to cool completely before chilling or freezing. The beans will keep for up to 1 week in the fridge or 1 month in the freezer.

If cooking from frozen, defrost overnight in the fridge. Reheat the beans in a saucepan over medium heat until bubbling.

Homemade
Takeaways

Homemade Takeaways

By the end of the week, many of us are all done in. No wonder we are reaching for the phone to order in. Takeaways are a godsend but they can also crush your weekly budget.

With this plan, you can make your own homemade takeaways to stash away in the freezer for the next seven Friday nights. How good is that?! How much will you save? It all adds up.

Menu

Turkish Pizzas

Lamb Rogan Josh

Thai Green Curry

Loaded Fried Rice

Teriyaki Chicken

Lemon Chicken

Burgers with Bacon & Cheese

Shopping List

Meat & Fish

700 g boneless lamb shoulder
200 g lamb mince
3.6 kg chicken thighs, boneless
1.5 kg chicken breasts
200 g small prawns or shrimp
14 bacon rashers
600 g good quality beef mince

Fruit & Veg

5 onions
2 heads garlic
1 lettuce
2 tomatoes
13 cm piece ginger
3 carrots
2 celery stalks
2 corn cobs
2 red capsicums
2 handfuls green beans
5 spring onions
4 handfuls baby spinach
2 large red chillies
2 bunches coriander
1 bunch Thai or regular basil
3 kaffir lime leaves (optional)
2½ lemons

Dairy & Frozen

100 ml plain yoghurt
6 eggs
100 g mozzarella
100 g feta
1 cup frozen peas
butter (for burger buns)
150 g sliced cheese

Tins, Jars & Dry Goods

2½ cups basmati rice
3 x 400 g tins diced tomatoes
1 x 400 ml tin coconut milk

Pantry Essentials

canola, sunflower or grapeseed oil
olive oil
oil, for frying
1 cup chicken stock
650 g flour
½ tsp baking powder
½ cup plus 1 tbs cornflour
2 tsp dry active yeast
⅓ cup plus 1 tsp caster sugar
1 tbs brown sugar
2 tbs honey
1 tbs tomato paste
salt
pepper
white pepper

mayonnaise
tomato sauce (ketchup)
mustard
3 tsp fish sauce
⅓ cup mirin
⅓ cup soy sauce
3 tsp sweet paprika
1 tsp smoked paprika
3 tsp turmeric
1 tbs plus 1 tsp ground coriander
2 tsp ground cumin
1 tsp ground cardamom
1 tsp garam masala
1 cinnamon stick
½ tsp ground cinnamon

Other Ingredients

2 tablespoons dry sherry (or dry white wine)
10 burger buns

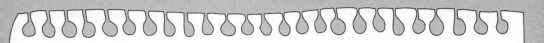

Serving Size

Each meal serves a family of 4 (approximately)

Preparation time

4 hours

Equipment

Preparation: sharp knives, chopping boards, measuring cups and spoons, kitchen scales, grater, sharp knives, rolling pin, food processor, citrus zester and juicer, edged baking tray, baking trays or pizza trays (optional), mortar and pestle (optional).

Cooking: ovenproof casserole dish or Dutch oven, heavy-based frying pan or wok, saucepans, rice cooker (optional).

Storage: large zip lock bags (optional), airtight containers suitable for freezing, foil.

Storage & Reheating

All of these meals are freezer-friendly and will keep for 1–2 months in the freezer. They should be defrosted the night before you plan to eat them, but don't panic if you only remember the following morning; just defrost them on the kitchen bench until dinnertime and then reheat fully.

Although most of these dishes will also keep for 1 week in the fridge, the Burgers with Bacon & Cheese are best eaten within two days of preparation. This is because homemade burgers made with fresh beef mince lack the preservatives that store-bought burgers contain. Unless frozen, raw beef mince actually has the shortest life-span of all meats. The burgers can be frozen when uncooked or cooked – just keep the accompaniments in the fridge until you're ready to eat the meal.

Once-A-Week Cooking Preparation

	Total	Turkish Pizzas	Lamb Rogan Josh	Thai Green Curry
Dough				
Pizza dough		prepare the dough and set aside to rise for 1½–2 hours		
Fresh Produce				
Onions	5	1 finely chopped	3 quartered	1 quartered
Garlic	2	3 cloves, finely chopped	5 cloves, roughly chopped	3 cloves, roughly chopped
Ginger	13 cm piece		4 cm piece, finely chopped	4 cm piece, roughly chopped
Carrots	3			
Celery	2 stalks			
Corn	2			
Capsicums	2		1 deseeded and quartered	1 thinly sliced
Green beans (handfuls)	2			2 handfuls, topped and tailed
Red chillies	2		2 large, deseeded and roughly chopped	
Spring onions	5			
Coriander	2		1 bunch, stalks thinly sliced, leaves roughly chopped	1 bunch, stalks thinly sliced, leaves roughly chopped
Basil	1			1 bunch, leaves picked
Lemon	2½	1 zested and 1½ juiced		
Tomato, lettuce	2, 1			
Cheese				
Mozzarella	100 g	100 g, grated		
Feta	100 g	100 g, crumbled		
Cheese	150 g			
Meat & Fish				
Boneless lamb shoulder	700 g		700 g, cut into 3 cm pieces	
Chicken thighs	3.6 kg			1.5 kg, cut into bite-sized pieces
Chicken breasts	1.5 kg			
Prawns or shrimp	200 g			
Bacon	14			

Loaded Fried Rice	Teriyaki Chicken	Lemon Chicken	Burgers with Bacon & Cheese
2 cloves, finely chopped	1 clove, smashed		
4 cm piece, finely chopped	1 cm piece, chopped		
3 finely diced			
2 stalks, finely diced			
2 cobs, kernels stripped			
5 tops, thinly sliced			
		1 juiced	
			prepare as you like just before serving burgers
			150 g, sliced
600 g cut into bite-sized pieces	1.5 kg, each thigh cut into 6 pieces		
		1.5 kg, cut into bite-sized pieces	
200 g, peeled			
4 rashers, thinly sliced			

Once-A-Week Cooking Plan

1. Prepare the pizza dough for the **Turkish Pizzas** and set aside to rise for 1½–2 hours.

2. On the stovetop, place an ovenproof casserole dish for the **Lamb Rogan Josh**, a heavy-based frying pan or wok for the **Loaded Fried Rice** and a large saucepan for the **Thai Green Curry**.

3. Make the burgers for the **Burgers with Bacon & Cheese**. Freeze, or set aside in the fridge if planning to cook them within 2 days. You will make the burgers now and assemble on the day of eating.

4. Marinate the lamb for the **Lamb Rogan Josh**. Set aside for 1 hour.

5. Cook the rice for the **Loaded Fried Rice**. Set aside to cool.

6. Preheat the oven to 200°C.

7. Prepare and cook the **Thai Green Curry**.

8. Finish preparing the **Lamb Rogan Josh** and cook for 2 hours.

9. Marinate the chicken for the **Teriyaki Chicken** and set aside.

10. Prepare the toppings for the **Turkish Pizzas**.

11. Coat and fry the chicken for the **Lemon Chicken** and drain on paper towel. Mix the ingredients for the sauce except the cornflour and set aside to finish just before the end of cooking.

12. Cook the **Loaded Fried Rice** and set aside to cool.

13. Prepare the Teriyaki sauce and cook the **Teriyaki Chicken**.

14. Finally, roll out the dough for the **Turkish Pizzas**. Add the toppings and bake.

15. Allow all dishes to cool completely before chilling or freezing.

Turkish Pizzas

Ingredients

Dough

650 g plain flour

1 teaspoon salt

3 tablespoons olive oil

2 teaspoons dry active yeast

390 ml warm water

Meat Topping

1 tablespoon olive oil

1 onion, finely chopped

1 garlic clove, finely chopped

200 g lamb mince

1 teaspoon smoked paprika

½ teaspoon ground cinnamon

½ teaspoon salt

1 tablespoon brown sugar

1 tablespoon tomato paste

Vegetable Topping

2 teaspoons olive oil

2 garlic cloves, finely chopped

4 handfuls baby spinach

zest of 1 lemon

juice of 1½ lemons

100 g feta, crumbled

100 g mozzarella, grated

Method

1. To make the dough, place the flour, salt and olive oil in the bowl of a stand mixer or large bowl.
2. In a separate jug or bowl, add the yeast to the warm water and set aside for 10 minutes until the mixture begins to froth. Pour into the flour and mix until a rough dough forms. If you are using a stand mixer, knead the dough for 10 minutes. Alternatively, if you are making the dough by hand, scrape the dough onto a well-floured surface and knead for 10 minutes.
3. Scrape the dough into a large lightly oiled bowl. Cover with plastic wrap. Set aside for at least 1–1½ hours or until doubled in size.
4. To make the vegetable topping, heat the olive oil in a medium-sized saucepan over medium heat. Add the garlic and sauté until starting to colour. Add the spinach and stir for a few minutes until wilted.

Remove from the heat and set aside to cool. Add the lemon zest and two-thirds of the lemon juice.

5. Combine the feta and mozzarella in a small bowl. Add the spinach mixture and set aside.

6. To make the meat topping, heat the olive oil in the same saucepan over medium heat and sauté the onion and garlic. When the onions are lightly golden, add the mince and turn the heat up to high. Cook, stirring frequently, until the meat is well browned with crisp edges. Add the spices, sugar and salt and stir to combine. When the spices become aromatic, add the tomato paste and cook off for 5 minutes. Remove from the heat.

7. Preheat the oven to 200°C.

8. On a well-floured work surface, divide the dough into four pieces and roll out into rough oval shapes. Place each pizza base on a greased baking tray or pizza tray. Spread the vegetable mixture on two bases and the meat mixture on the remaining bases.

9. Bake in the oven for about 15–20 minutes or until the pizza edges are golden and the underside is cooked.

10. Drizzle over the remaining lemon juice before serving.

Serving Suggestion
Serve with a crunchy green salad.

Storage & Reheating
Allow to cool completely before chilling or freezing. Wrap well with plastic wrap and store for up to 1 week in the fridge or 1 month in the freezer.

To cook from frozen, partially defrost the pizzas for 10 minutes then reheat in a 200°C oven for 10–15 minutes, or until warmed through and golden brown on top.

Lamb Rogan Josh

This is a lovely mild curry for everyone in the family to enjoy.

Ingredients

5 garlic cloves, roughly chopped

4 cm piece ginger, finely chopped

100 ml plain yoghurt

1 teaspoon turmeric

1 teaspoon pepper

700 g boneless lamb shoulder, cut into 3 cm pieces

3 onions, quartered

1 red capsicum, deseeded and quartered

2 large red chillies, deseeded and roughly chopped

1 bunch coriander, stalks thinly sliced, leaves roughly chopped

1 tablespoon ground coriander

1 teaspoon ground cumin

1 teaspoon ground cardamom

1 cinnamon stick

2 tablespoons canola, sunflower or grapeseed oil

3 teaspoons sweet paprika

3 x 400 g tins diced tomatoes

1 teaspoon salt

Method

1. Combine the garlic, ginger, yoghurt, turmeric and pepper in a large bowl. Add the lamb and stir to coat. Set aside to marinate for 1 hour.
2. Preheat the oven to 180°C.
3. Combine the onion, red capsicum, chilli and coriander stalks in a food processor and process into a smooth paste.
4. Place a casserole dish or Dutch oven over a medium–high heat and toast the coriander, cardamom, cinnamon stick and cumin until fragrant, about 1 minute. Add the oil and the curry paste and cook, stirring frequently, for 5–7 minutes. Add the tinned tomatoes, sweet paprika, marinated lamb and 200 ml water. Stir to combine, then bring to the boil and season with the salt.
5. Put the lid on, transfer the dish to the oven. Cook for 2 hours. Season to taste and serve, garnished with the chopped coriander leaves.

Serving Suggestion

Serve the curry with basmati rice on the side and a dollop of cooling yoghurt.

Storage & Reheating

Allow to cool completely before chilling or freezing. The curry will keep for up to 1 week in the fridge or 1 month in the freezer.

If cooking from frozen, defrost overnight in the fridge. Preheat the oven to 180°C and reheat thoroughly in an ovenproof dish with a lid. Smaller portions can be reheated in the microwave or on the stovetop.

Thai Green Curry

Ingredients

1 onion, quartered

3 garlic cloves, roughly chopped

4 cm piece ginger, roughly chopped

1 bunch coriander, stalks thinly sliced, leaves roughly chopped, for garnish

2 teaspoons ground turmeric

1 teaspoon ground coriander

1 teaspoon ground cumin

1 teaspoon garam masala

2 tablespoons canola, sunflower or grapeseed oil

1 x 400 ml tin coconut milk

3 teaspoons fish sauce

1 teaspoon caster sugar

1.5 kg chicken thighs, boneless, cut into bite-sized pieces

3 kaffir lime leaves (optional)

1 red capsicum, thinly sliced

2 handfuls green beans, topped and tailed

1 bunch Thai or regular basil, leaves picked, for garnish

Method

1. Place the onion, garlic, ginger and coriander stalks in a food processor and process until you have a smooth paste. Alternatively, pound the ingredients in a mortar and pestle.

2. Place a large saucepan over medium–high heat and toast the spices for 1 minute, until fragrant. Add the oil and curry paste and cook, stirring frequently, for 5 minutes or until fragrant. Add the coconut milk, fish sauce and sugar and bring to the boil, then reduce to a simmer.

3. Add the chicken and cook for 8–10 minutes. If using, crumple the kaffir lime leaves in your hands to release their aroma and add to the pan. Add the capsicum and beans and simmer for 2 minutes. Garnish with the reserved coriander and the basil leaves.

Serving Suggestion

Serve with steamed jasmine rice and lime wedges.

Storage & Reheating

Allow to cool completely before chilling or freezing. The curry will keep for up to 1 week in the fridge or 2 months in the freezer.

If cooking from frozen, defrost overnight in the fridge. Reheat thoroughly in a large saucepan on the stovetop.

Loaded Fried Rice

Ingredients

2½ cups basmati rice

3 tablespoons canola, sunflower or grapeseed oil

4 eggs, beaten

4 cm piece ginger, finely chopped

2 garlic cloves, finely chopped

3 carrots, finely diced

2 celery stalks, finely diced

600 g chicken thighs, boneless, cut into bite-sized pieces

4 bacon rashers, thinly sliced

2 corn cobs, kernels stripped

1 cup frozen peas

200 g small prawns, peeled

5 spring onions, tops only, thinly sliced

2 teaspoons soy sauce

3 teaspoons mirin

½ teaspoon white pepper

Method

1. Place the rice in a large saucepan with 3¾ cups water. Cover, and bring to the boil over medium–high heat. Reduce the heat to low and simmer for 18 minutes. Remove from the heat and set aside for 5 minutes before fluffing the rice with a fork. Alternatively, cook the rice in a rice cooker.

2. Spread the rice on a large baking tray. Set aside in the fridge to dry out and cool.

3. Heat 2 tablespoons of the oil in a large, heavy-based non-stick frying pan or wok over medium heat. Pour in the egg and season with a pinch of salt. Cook for 3–4 minutes, then flip and cook for a further 1 minute. Slide the omelette onto a plate and set aside.

4. Add the remaining oil, ginger and garlic to the frying pan or wok and sauté until the garlic begins to colour. Add the carrot and celery and cook, stirring frequently, for 8 minutes.

5. Add the chicken and bacon and cook for 7 minutes until the bacon is crisp and the chicken is starting to brown. Add the prawns, spring onions, corn, peas, dried rice, soy sauce, mirin and white pepper. Stir and cook for 5 minutes.

6. Dice the omelette and return to the pan. Stir to combine and adjust the seasoning, if necessary.

Storage & Reheating

Allow to cool completely before chilling or freezing. The fried rice will keep for up to 3 days in the fridge or 1 month in the freezer.

If cooking from frozen, defrost overnight in the fridge. Toss in a hot wok with a little oil until heated through.

Teriyaki Chicken

Ingredients

1.5 kg chicken thighs, boneless, cut into 6 pieces each

¼ cup soy sauce plus an additional 1 tablespoon

¼ cup mirin plus an additional 1 tablespoon

1 tablespoon honey

1 garlic clove, smashed

1 cm piece ginger, chopped

1 tablespoon canola, sunflower or grapeseed oil

Method

1. Combine the chicken with the 1 tablespoon of soy sauce and mirin in a large bowl and set aside.
2. Combine the remaining soy sauce, mirin, honey, smashed garlic clove and ginger in a small saucepan. Bring to a simmer and stir to dissolve the honey. Simmer for 5 minutes until the sauce is thick and sticky. Remove from the heat and set aside.
3. Heat the oil in a large frying pan over medium heat. Add the chicken and cook for 5–8 minutes or until cooked through. Add the teriyaki sauce and simmer for 1–2 minutes.

Serving Suggestion

Serve with steamed rice, chopped cucumber and sliced cabbage on the side.

Storage & Reheating

Allow to cool completely before chilling or freezing. The teriyaki chicken will keep for up to 1 week in the fridge or 2 months in the freezer.

If cooking from frozen, defrost overnight in the fridge. Reheat thoroughly in the microwave or on the stovetop.

Lemon Chicken

Ingredients

2 tablespoons dry sherry or white wine

1 tablespoon soy sauce

1 teaspoon salt

1.5 kg chicken breasts, cut into bite-sized pieces

2 eggs

½ cup cornflour

½ teaspoon baking powder

2 cups vegetable or rice bran oil, for frying

Sauce

1 cup chicken stock

⅓ cup sugar

juice of 1 lemon

2 tablespoons canola, sunflower or grapeseed oil

1 tablespoon cornflour

Method

1. Combine the sherry, soy sauce and salt in a large bowl or large zip lock bag. Add the chicken and toss to coat in the sauce. Set aside to marinate for 30 minutes.
2. In another bowl, whisk the eggs, half of the cornflour and the baking powder to make a batter.
3. Heat the oil in a heavy-based saucepan to 180°C, or until a cube of bread dropped into the oil turns brown in 15 seconds. Dip the chicken pieces in the batter before dropping into the hot oil. Deep-fry for 2–3 minutes until golden. Remove from the oil and drain on paper towel.

★ **At this point, once cool, the chicken can be chilled or frozen until needed.**

4. To make the sauce, combine all of the ingredients except the cornflour in a small bowl and chill for 30 minutes.
5. Transfer the sauce to a small saucepan, add the cornflour and simmer for 3 minutes until the sauce is clear and thickened. Pour the lemon sauce over the fried chicken and serve.

Serving Suggestion

Serve with steamed rice and a green salad on the side.

Storage & Reheating

Allow the deep-fried chicken to cool completely before chilling or freezing. This will keep for up to 4 months in the freezer and 3 days in the fridge.

If cooking from frozen, defrost overnight in the fridge. Re-fry the chicken in 2 tablespoons of oil and follow steps 4–5 to complete making the dish.

You can freeze the Lemon Sauce, omitting the cornflour, in a zip lock bag. To reheat, allow to defrost in the fridge overnight then stir through cornflour when cooking.

Burgers with Bacon & Cheese

These burgers are super easy and only take 20 minutes to make.

Ingredients

600 g good quality beef mince

2½ teaspoons salt

1 teaspoon pepper

150 g sliced cheese

3 tablespoons butter

10 burger buns, cut in half

10 bacon rashers

1 lettuce, shredded

2 tomatoes, sliced

mayonnaise, for spreading

tomato sauce (ketchup), for
    spreading

mustard, for spreading

Method

1. Combine the mince, salt and pepper in a large bowl. Gently
    shape the meat into 10 patties. Do not press too firmly or the patties
    will be tough.

★   **At this point, you can chill or freeze the patties.**

2. Preheat the oven to 170°C or a BBQ to medium.
3. Cook the patties for 2–3 minutes before flipping and placing a
    cheese slice on top of each one. Cook for a further 2–3 minutes or
    until cooked to your liking.
4. Butter the insides of the burger buns and toast in the oven or on the
    BBQ for 4–5 minutes. Fry or BBQ the bacon until crisp.
5. Place a burger on the bottom half of each bun. Top with a
    bacon rasher, a few lettuce leaves and a slice of tomato. Spread
    the mayonnaise, tomato sauce and mustard (or your preferred
    combination) on the undersides of the bun tops and serve.

Storage & Reheating

The uncooked patties will keep for 2 days in the fridge. The
accompaniments will keep for up to 1 week. Cooked burgers can
be frozen for up to 3 months and refrigerated for up to 4 days.

If cooking from frozen, defrost overnight in the fridge, then
follow steps 2–5 to cook.

Sickness Recovery Meals

Sickness Recovery Meals

When you've had a bout of the dreaded gastro in your family, small meals that are gentle on the stomach are the way to go. This menu is designed with that in mind and so is a little different to our other plans. We have increased the quantities and decreased the variety of the meals, so that there is enough for dinners and lunches.

We've designed this plan so that meals are easy to pull together, so if you're sick too, the cooking is easy and you can pass out afterwards.

Alternatively, if someone you know or a local family in the neighbourhood is feeling poorly, nurture them by cooking up one of these dishes. They will be eternally grateful!

Menu

Healing Chicken Soup

Lemon & Thyme Chicken Breasts

Steamed Asparagus, Cauliflower
& Green Vegetables

Grapefruit, Orange & Pineapple Fruit Salad

Honey Ginger Syrup

Shopping List

Meat & Fish	Fruit & Veg
3 kg chicken breasts	3 onions 3 heads garlic 16 cm piece ginger 8 carrots 1 bunch celery 2 bunches asparagus 1 head cauliflower 2 heads broccoli 1 bunch English spinach 1 bunch silverbeet or kale 1 bunch spring onions 1 bunch thyme 1 bunch coriander 6 lemons 4 large pink or ruby grapefruit 4 large oranges 1 pineapple
Tins, Jars & Dry Goods	**Pantry Essentials**
none	olive oil 10.25 litres chicken stock 1 cup honey 1 tbs cider vinegar 3 tbs sugar white pepper salt ½ cup plus 2 tsp soy sauce 4 star anise

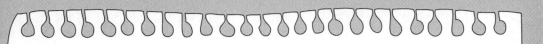

Serving Size

Each meal serves a family of 4 (approximately) for lunch and dinner – please see earlier note.

Preparation time

1½ hours

Equipment

Large stockpot, large baking dishes, 8 microwave-safe, zip lock bags or containers.

Serving Suggestions with Sickness Recovery Plans

Because of the nature of this plan, we recommend you serve the meals with plain rice and/or noodles with the Healing Chicken Soup, Lemon & Thyme Chicken Breasts and Steamed Asparagus, Cauliflower & Green Vegetables. But of course, see how you feel and what everyone feels up to.

Storage & Reheating

All of the meals in this plan can be kept in the fridge for up to 1 week. Individual serves can be reheated as required.

Apart from the Grapefruit, Orange & Pineapple Fruit Salad and the Honey Ginger Syrup, all meals can be frozen and consumed at a later date. See individual recipes for freezing instructions.

To reduce handling and risk of contamination, we recommend decanting the chicken soup into smaller containers rather than two large ones.

Once-A-Week Cooking Preparation

	Total	Healing Chicken Soup	Lemon & Thyme Chicken Breasts	Steamed Asparagus, Cauliflower & Green Vegetables
Fresh Produce				
Onion	3	3 finely chopped		
Garlic	3	1 head, cloves peeled	1 head, finely chopped	5 cloves, finely chopped
Ginger	16 cm	8 cm piece, sliced		4 cm piece, finely chopped
Carrots	8	8 finely diced		
Celery	1	1 bunch, finely diced		
Thyme	1		1 bunch, leaves picked and chopped	
Spring onions	1	1 bunch, white ends reserved, green tops thinly sliced		
Coriander	1	1 bunch, stalks finely chopped, leaves roughly chopped		
Asparagus	2			2 bunches, woody ends removed, spears cut in half
Cauliflower	1			1 head, cut into florets
Broccoli	2			2 heads, cut into florets, stem peeled and cut into batons
Silverbeet or kale	1			1 bunch, stems removed, leaves roughly chopped
English spinach	1			1 bunch, stems removed, leaves roughly chopped
Grapefruit	4			
Oranges	4			
Pineapple	1			
Lemons	6		1 zested and juiced 1 zested, peeled and chopped	
Meat				
Chicken breasts	3 kg	1.5 kg, reserved	1.5 kg, butterflied	

Grapefruit, Orange & Pineapple Fruit Salad	Honey Ginger Syrup
	4 cm piece, finely grated
4 peeled and cut into bite-sized pieces	
4 peeled and cut into bite-sized pieces	
1 peeled, core removed, flesh cut into bite-sized pieces	
	4 juiced

Once-A-Week Cooking Plan

1. Start with the **Healing Chicken Soup**, as this has the longest preparation time.

2. Make the **Honey Ginger Syrup**, then set aside to cool.

3. Preheat the oven to 200°C.

4. Prepare the **Lemon & Thyme Chicken Breasts** and place in the oven.

5. Prepare the **Steamed Asparagus, Cauliflower & Green Vegetables** and the **Grapefruit, Orange & Pineapple Fruit Salad**.

6. Allow all dishes to cool completely before chilling or freezing.

Healing Chicken Soup

Serves 20–25

This super simple, shortcut version of the MamaBake Healing Chicken Soup recipe will combat even the gnarliest of bugs! In our usual recipe, we use a whole chicken but because you might be unwell too, we've opted for chicken breasts to make it as simple as possible.

Ingredients

10 litres chicken stock

4 star anise

1 garlic bulb, cloves peeled

8 cm piece ginger, sliced

1 bunch spring onions, white ends reserved, green tops thinly sliced

1 bunch coriander, stalks finely chopped, leaves roughly chopped

1.5 kg chicken breasts

3 onions, finely chopped

8 carrots, finely diced

1 bunch celery, finely diced

½ cup soy sauce

3 tablespoons sugar

½ teaspoon white pepper

Method

1. Place the stock, star anise, garlic, ginger, coriander stalks and spring onion ends in a large stockpot and bring to the boil over high heat. Reduce the heat to low and add the chicken breasts. Cover, and simmer for 15 minutes or until the chicken is cooked through. Remove from the heat.
2. Remove the chicken from the stock and set aside. Return the stock to the boil, then add the onion, carrot, celery, soy sauce, sugar and white pepper. Reduce the heat to low and simmer for 40 minutes.
3. Shred the chicken meat and return to the pan along with the sliced spring onion and coriander leaves. Season, to taste.

Serving Suggestion

Serve with noodles or a side of steamed white rice.

Storage & Reheating

Allow to cool completely before chilling or freezing. If refrigerating, keep in individual containers or 2 large containers and ladle out serves to reheat as necessary.

The soup will keep for up to 1 week in the fridge and 2–3 months in the freezer.

If cooking from frozen, defrost overnight in the fridge. Reheat single or multiple servings in the microwave or on the stovetop until just simmering. The reheated soup should not be stored again.

Lemon & Thyme Chicken Breasts

12 serves

Ingredients

½ cup olive oil

1 garlic bulb, finely chopped

1 bunch thyme, leaves picked and chopped

1 cup chicken stock

1 tablespoon cider vinegar

zest of 2 lemons

juice of 1 lemon

1 lemon, peeled and roughly chopped

1.5 kg chicken breasts, butterflied

1½ teaspoons salt

black pepper, to taste

Method

1. Preheat the oven to 200°C.
2. Heat the olive oil in a small saucepan over low heat. Add the garlic and thyme and sauté for 1 minute, then remove from the heat. Add the stock, cider vinegar, lemon zest, lemon juice and the salt. Stir to combine, then pour into a large baking dish.
3. Place the chicken in the dish in one layer without any overlapping (you may need to cut the chicken into smaller pieces to achieve this). Spoon the sauce over the chicken and season with black pepper. Tuck the chopped lemon in between the chicken.
4. Bake for 25–30 minutes or until the chicken is lightly browned and the meat bounces back when firmly pressed in the centre. Remove from the oven and set aside to rest for at least 10 minutes.

Serving Suggestion

Serve with a side of steamed white rice.

Storage & Reheating

Allow to cool completely before chilling or freezing. The chicken will keep for up to 1 week in the fridge or 2 months in the freezer.

If cooking from frozen, defrost overnight in the fridge. Reheat individual serves in the microwave or on the stovetop as required. Defrosted, reheated chicken should not be stored again.

Steamed Asparagus, Cauliflower & Green Vegetables

8 serves

Ingredients

2 bunches asparagus, woody ends removed, spears cut in half

1 head cauliflower, cut into florets

2 heads broccoli, cut into florets, stem peeled and cut into batons

1 bunch silverbeet or kale, stems removed, leaves roughly chopped

1 bunch English spinach, stems removed, leaves roughly chopped

5 garlic cloves, finely chopped

4 cm piece ginger, finely chopped

2 teaspoons soy sauce

Method

1. Combine all of the ingredients in a large bowl. Divide the mixture into 8 microwave-safe zip lock bags or containers. If you don't use a microwave, keep all the vegetables in a large zip lock bag or container and steam individual serves.

2. Steam the vegetables in the microwave or in a steamer on the stovetop.

Serving Suggestion

Serve with plain noodles.

Storage & Reheating

This dish will keep for up to 1 week in the fridge or 1 month in the freezer. There is no need to defrost the vegetables before cooking.

Grapefruit, Orange & Pineapple Fruit Salad

8 serves

This is a light, fresh snack for the road to recovery.

Ingredients

4 large pink or ruby grapefruit, peeled and cut into bite-sized pieces

4 large oranges, peeled and cut into bite-sized pieces

1 pineapple, peeled, core removed, flesh cut into bite-sized pieces

Method

Combine the fruit and refrigerate in an airtight container.

Storage

The fruit will keep for up to 1 week in the fridge and should not be frozen.

Honey Ginger Syrup

1 cup

Ingredients

1 cup honey

4 cm piece ginger, finely grated

juice of 4 lemons

Method

1. Combine the honey and 1 cup water in a medium-sized saucepan. Bring the mixture to the boil and simmer until the liquid begins to thicken. Remove from the heat and add the ginger. Set aside to infuse for about 1 hour.
2. Strain the syrup through a fine-meshed sieve and pour into a jar or other container.
3. Combine 1 teaspoon of the syrup with lemon juice, to taste, and add hot water.

Storage

Allow to cool completely before chilling. Store in a tightly sealed glass jar in the fridge for 3–5 months. Do not freeze the syrup.

Pizza Bases, Rolls, Bread & Flatbreads

Pizza Bases, Rolls, Bread & Flatbreads

Nothing says home like the smell of freshly baked bread and there is something hugely satisfying in baking your own and seeing the end result.

Once you get the hang of producing this amount of bread dough, you can vary what you make with it. This recipe is a great starting point for anything bread-based! Let your imagination run wild.

For example, you could replace the pizza bases and make extra rolls flavoured with different herbs and seeds; or you could make more loaves and fewer rolls and flatbreads. It's all up to you.

But for the moment, and particularly if you're starting out and are a bit shy of bread-making, these recipes and quantities are great to show you what you can achieve.

Menu

4 Large Pizza Bases

25 Bread Rolls

3 Large Bread Loaves

20 Flatbreads

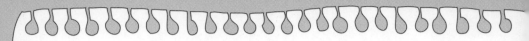

Shopping List

Pantry Essentials

5 kg flour (half wholemeal mixed with
    half bread flour works really well),
    plus extra for dusting and kneading
100 g salt
3 litres warm water
50 g dry active yeast
olive oil

Serving Size

Makes 5 batches of dough.

Preparation time

5–6 hours (including proving time).

Equipment

Preparation: stand mixer (optional but really useful! Or some extra sets of hands and a large helping of elbow grease!), 5 large metal or glass bowls, measuring spoons, measuring jug.
Cooking: baking trays, pizza trays.
Storage: plastic wrap or foil.

Storage & Reheating

Bread will keep for about 1 week in an airtight container out of the fridge. Refrigerated and well wrapped, it will keep for up to 2 weeks. Pizza bases don't refrigerate well and should be frozen until needed.

All unbaked and baked bread can be frozen, well wrapped. Unbaked bread can be kept for 2–3 months in the freezer. Baked bead can be kept for 6 months in the freezer. When freezing bread, wrap tightly in freezer-proof plastic bags or plastic wrap and foil.

Flavour Ideas

Once you get the hang of making bread, you can have a lot of fun adding interesting textures and flavours to your flatbreads, rolls, pizza bases and loaves. If this is your first crack at making bread, don't worry too much about including extra ingredients (although if you're a Recipe Daredevil Adventurer – go for it!). Optional extras might include seeds, spices, herbs, nuts, grated cheeses – basically any combination you like.

- **Cheesy Pizza Bases:** Combine 100 g grated mozzarella with 50 g grated parmesan and add to your bases before cooking for an extra-cheesy crust.

- **Cheesy Ham Rolls**: Top bread rolls with 300 g grated tasty cheese and 200 g diced ham.

- **White Bap Rolls:** Get the bap effect by dusting your rolls in white flour before baking.

- **Chia & Pumpkin Seed Flatbreads, Rolls or Loaves:** Add 2 tablespoons of chia seeds and 3 tablespoons of pumpkin seeds to your flatbreads, rolls or loaves (double the amount) at step 3 of the Once-A-Week Cooking Plan to make your bread even more wholesome and add some crunch!

- **Herb Bread:** Finely chop the leaves from 4 sprigs of rosemary and 4 sprigs of thyme and add them to flatbreads, pizza bases or loaves at step 3 of the Once-A-Week Cooking Plan.

- **Cinnamon Scroll Buns:** instead of rolling your bread roll batch into balls, roll the whole dough into one long rectangle about 1 cm thick. Spread with 80–100 g melted butter and sprinkle over 1 tablespoon of cinnamon combined with ½–¾ cup of brown sugar. Roll up tightly to make a long sausage. Cut the sausage into 16–25 pieces and bake, spiral side up, at 180°C for 20–25 minutes until golden and oozing.

- **Rich Fruit Loaf:** Add 100 g currants, 100 g sultanas, 50 g sliced dried apricot, 50 g pitted and sliced dates and 50 g sliced dried figs to your loaf dough at step 3 of the Once-A-Week Cooking Plan.

Once-A-Week Cooking Plan

Because this plan makes such a large batch of dough, it is best to divide the ingredients into 5 batches: each batch will have 1 kg of flour, 3½ teaspoons of yeast, 3½ teaspoons of salt and 600 ml warm water. Don't worry about washing the bowl in between batches.

1. Place the flour and salt in the bowl of a stand mixer or large bowl. Pour the warm water into a separate bowl and sprinkle the yeast on top. Set aside for 10 minutes until the mixture starts to froth.

2. Make a well in the centre of the flour and add the yeast and water. Mix until a rough dough forms with no loose flour at the bottom of the bowl. If using a stand mixer, knead for 6 minutes. Alternatively, if kneading by hand, transfer the dough to a well-floured work surface and knead for about 10 minutes or until a smooth elastic dough forms. (This is glorious, intense arm-working exercise; definitely the equivalent of an hour at the gym, but with the added bonus of homemade bread at the end!).

3. Add any extra ingredients (if you're being adventurous) here. Knead well to combine.

4. Place the dough ball in a lightly oiled large bowl and cover with plastic wrap. Set aside for 2 hours or until the dough has doubled in size. Repeat with the other batches of ingredients.

Pizza bases

1. Divide 1 batch of dough into 4 equal-sized pieces. On a well-dusted work surface, roll the dough into circles about 1½ cm thick.
2. Place the pizza bases on liberally floured thin baking trays or pizza trays. Dust each pizza base with flour and set aside to rise for a further 30 minutes. (Start making the bread rolls at this point).
3. Preheat the oven to 180°C.
4. Bake the pizza bases for 20 minutes or until just cooked in the centre but not coloured. Remove from the oven and set aside to cool.

Bread rolls

1. Divide 1 batch of dough into 25 equal-sized pieces and roll with a cupped hand into a ball. Transfer to two baking trays, spacing the dough 6 cm apart. Set aside to rest for a further 30 minutes, covered, or until the pizza bases are cooked. (Start making the bread loaves at this point).
2. Bake the rolls at 180°C for 25–30 minutes or until golden brown. Tap the bottom of the buns – they should sound hollow inside.
3. Once the rolls are cooked, increase the oven temperature to 200°C.

Bread loaves

1. Combine 2 batches of dough before dividing into 3 equal-sized pieces. Shape each piece into oval rounds. Transfer to a thin baking tray and slash each loaf in a cross-shaped pattern with a sharp knife. This helps the bread to expand.
2. Set aside to rest for a further 30 minutes, covered.
3. Bake for 45–60 minutes or until the bread is dark–golden brown all over and hollow-sounding when tapped underneath.

Flatbreads

1. Divide 1 batch of dough into 20 equal-sized pieces. Roll each piece into a rough oval, about 1 cm thick.
2. To cook on the stovetop, heat a griddle pan or non-stick frying pan over medium–high heat. Dry-fry each flatbread for 2 minutes on each side. When the bread bubbles and puffs up, it's time to flip it.

Storage

Allow all breads to cool completely (several hours for the large bread loaves) before chilling or freezing. The bread loaves can be sliced and then frozen, so slices can be defrosted as desired. Keep one loaf out to be consumed the week ahead. The rolls and flatbreads should be stored in zip lock bags before chilling or freezing. The pizza bases should be well wrapped with plastic wrap before chilling or freezing.

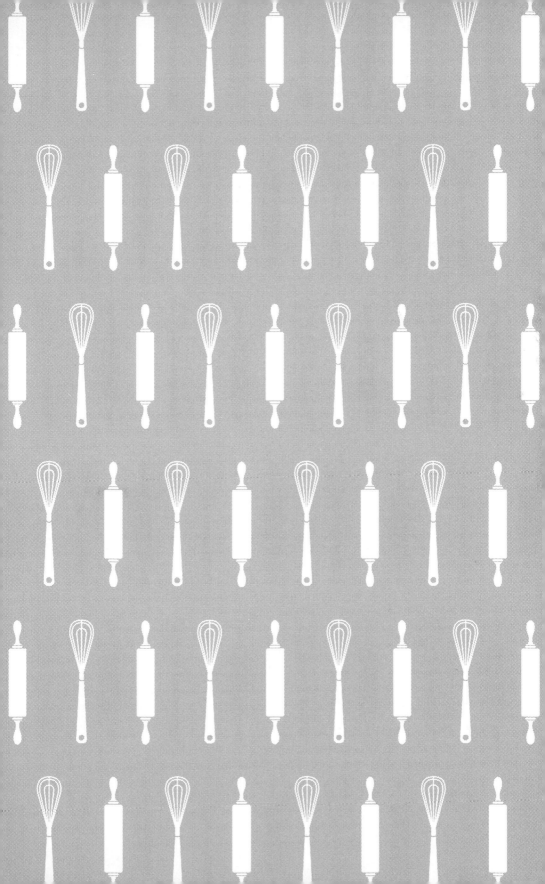

Part 2:
Big Batch Recipes

Big Batch Recipes

MamaBake is the home of big batch cooking either with other mums or if you're simply trying to get ahead for the week.

If you are MamaBaking with other mums this chapter will give you a great range of recipes to choose from. You can then either cook it up before you go the session so that you can enjoy a relaxed cuppa or you can cook it at the time with the other women – which is always so much more fun than cooking alone.

Cooking in bulk means you can have meals in the freezer ready to reheat for those evenings when you haven't got a thing left in the tank to drag out yet another dinner. And you'll be saving on takeaways too.

See each recipe for Storage and Reheating instructions.

Big Batch
Savoury Dishes

Butter Chicken

Serves approximately 12 people or
approximately 4 families of 4

This is an old, old favourite of MamaBakers across the world. It is very popular and very easy to make. The fragrance from the spices fills your home and it is a pleasure to cook and share with family and friends. We have found that this recipe is a universal hit with kids everywhere too.

Ingredients

6 tablespoons peanut oil

3 kg boneless chicken thigh, quartered or halved

180 g ghee or butter

6 teaspoons garam masala

5 teaspoons sweet paprika

6 teaspoons ground coriander

3 tablespoons finely chopped fresh ginger

¾ teaspoon chilli powder

3 cinnamon sticks

18 cardamom pods, lightly crushed

1 litre passata (puréed tomatoes)

3 tablespoons sugar

¾ cup plain yoghurt

1½ cups cream

3 tablespoons lemon juice

Method

1. Heat a little of the oil in a large wok over a medium–high heat. Add the chicken in batches and stir-fry until browned (add extra oil as required). Transfer to a heatproof bowl and set aside.
2. Reduce the heat and add the ghee or butter to the wok until melted. Add the garam masala, sweet paprika, coriander, ginger, chilli powder, cinnamon sticks and cardamom pods and stir-fry until the fragrance fills the kitchen, about one minute.
3. Return the chicken to the wok and stir to coat in the spices for 1 minute. Add the passata and sugar and simmer, stirring frequently, for 15 minutes, or until the chicken is tender and the sauce has thickened.
4. Add the yoghurt, cream and lemon juice and simmer for a further 5 minutes or until the sauce has thickened slightly.

5. Remove the cinnamon sticks and cardamom pods before serving (they are a bitter surprise if you accidentally bite down on one!).

Serving Suggestions

Serve with steamed rice or naan bread on the side.

Note: You can add a couple of handfuls of chopped vegetables at step 3 to make the dish go further and to add some extra goodness to the proceedings.

Storage & Reheating

This dish can be frozen once cooked and cooled. Defrost overnight in the fridge and ensure that it is reheated slowly and thoroughly.

Cauliflower & Cheese Fritters

(gluten free)

Makes approximately 48 fritters

Ingredients

4 cauliflowers (about 1.4 kg), florets roughly chopped

400 g gluten-free, plain flour

16 eggs

400 g cheese (use a single cheese or a combination of your favourites), grated

4 teaspoons Dijon mustard

zest of 4 lemons

1 bunch flat-leaf parsley, roughly chopped

olive oil, for frying

Method

1. Working in batches, pulse the cauliflower in a food processor until it resembles rice grains. Heat a large pan over medium heat and, working in batches, dry-fry the cauliflower 'rice' for about 10 minutes or until just soft. Set aside to cool.

2. Place the flour in a large bowl and add the eggs, one at a time, whisking until the batter is smooth. Stir in the cheese, mustard, lemon zest and parsley. Stir through the cauliflower rice and season, to taste.

3. Heat a little olive oil in a heavy-based frying pan. Using a dessert spoon, scoop the mixture into patties and carefully lower them into the oil. You will need to cook the fritters in batches. Cook for 3–5 minutes, until the fritters are golden brown, then flip and cook for a further 3–5 minutes.

4. Remove from the heat and set aside on a plate while you repeat the process with the remaining mixture.

Serving Suggestion

Serve with steamed green vegetables and lemon wedges.

Storage & Reheating

The fritters can be frozen once cooked and cooled. Defrost overnight in the fridge and reheat thoroughly in a 180°C oven.

Cheese & Mustard Chicken Burgers

(gluten & grain free)

Makes approximately 16 burgers

Perfect for those 'can't be bothered' cooking nights, these one-bowl burgers are fantastic in the lunchbox the next day too.

Ingredients

1 kg chicken mince

2 onions, finely chopped

1 cup almond meal (or breadcrumbs if there are nut allergy issues)

2 tablespoons grain mustard

1½ cups finely chopped flat-leaf parsley

2 cups grated cheese (cheddar or your favourite hard cheese)

1 egg, lightly beaten

4 garlic cloves, crushed

olive oil for shallow-frying

Method

1. Combine all of the ingredients except the olive oil in a large mixing bowl. Using damp hands, shape the mixture into palm-sized patties.

★ You can freeze the uncooked patties at this stage.

2. Heat enough olive oil to cover the base of a heavy-based frying pan over medium heat. Working in batches, gently fry the patties, for a few minutes on each side, or until cooked through and golden. Transfer to a plate lined with paper towel and allow to cool a little.

Serving Suggestion

These are amazing served as is, with a simple side salad or, as a more traditional burger in a bun. The burgers can be eaten hot or cold.

Storage & Reheating

To freeze uncooked patties, layer between pieces of baking paper in an airtight container. To freeze cooked burgers, cool completely, then lay flat in a zip lock bag, or layer between baking paper and store in an airtight container.

Chicken Nuggets

Serves approximately 3 families, based on 4 nuggets per person

Homemade chicken nuggets are an absolute cinch to prepare! A great MamaBake dish to cook with children.

Ingredients

2 cups breadcrumbs

1 cup parsley, finely chopped (optional)

½ cup finely grated parmesan (optional)

1 kg chicken breasts or boneless chicken thighs, chopped into bite-sized cubes

4 eggs, beaten

Method

1. Preheat the oven to 200°C.
2. Place the breadcrumbs, herbs and cheese (if using) in a bowl and mix together. Season, to taste. Place the beaten egg in a separate bowl.
3. Dip the chicken into the egg, then roll in the breadcrumbs.

★ **The chicken nuggets can be frozen at this stage.**

4. Lay the crumbed chicken on a greased baking tray and cook for about 20 minutes or until golden, turning halfway through.

Serving Suggestion

Serve with mayonnaise thinned with the juice of 1 lemon, some homemade hot chips and salad.

Storage & Reheating

Nuggets can be frozen uncooked for approximately 30 minutes or until cooked through thoroughly, or once cooked and cooled. There is no need to defrost the nuggets – just cook or reheat in a 200°C oven.

Homemade Fried Chicken

Serves 4 families of 4

A budget-friendly recipe for the tastiest fried chicken you'll ever have!

Just to be clear: chicken ribs, if you haven't heard of them before, are not the actual ribs of a chicken but the shoulder meat area of the bird. You can get these at your local butchers.

Ingredients

⅔ cup soy sauce (or tamari for gluten free)

80 g sugar

4 kg chicken ribs

4 cups gluten-free potato starch or plain flour

2 tablespoons paprika

2 tablespoons garlic powder

3 teaspoons salt

2 teaspoons pepper

1 litre neutral oil such as rice bran or canola oil, for frying (oil can be cooled, strained and stored for future frying)

Method

1. Combine the soy sauce and sugar in a large bowl or divide between two bowls, if necessary, to fit the chicken. Toss the chicken in the marinade and set aside in the fridge for at least 2 hours or, preferably, overnight.

2. In another large bowl, combine the potato starch or plain flour, paprika, garlic powder, salt and pepper.

★ **At this point the coating can be stored in the pantry and the marinated chicken frozen.**

3. Bring the chicken to room temperature for 30 minutes. Toss the chicken in the spice mix, ensuring that each piece is thoroughly coated.

4. Heat the oil in a medium-sized heavy-based saucepan to 180°C. Test the temperature by dropping a cube of bread into the oil. If it turns golden brown in 15 seconds, it's ready. Adjust the temperature as necessary – oil that is not hot enough will result in soggy rather than crisp chicken; oil that is too hot will cook the outside of the chicken too quickly, leaving the inside undercooked.

5. Fry the ribs in batches of 4–5 pieces at a time for 2–3 minutes or until completely golden brown on both sides. Drain on a wire rack over a baking tray lined with paper towel. Repeat with the remaining ribs.
6. Serve immediately or allow to cool completely before dividing and freezing.

Serving Suggestion

These are lovely served with mashed potato and coleslaw, rice and green veggies or even with just some fresh bread and dipping sauce.

Storage & Reheating

Uncooked marinated chicken can be frozen. To cook, defrost the chicken completely and allow it to sit at room temperature for 30 minutes before coating and frying. Fried chicken can also be frozen once completely cool. Defrost overnight in the fridge before placing on a baking tray and reheating at 200°C for 15–20 minutes.

Frozen Pizzas

Makes 4 pizzas

When life is hectic, dinner can be as simple as heating the oven and throwing in a homemade frozen pizza, leaving you free to unwind and relax with one less 'to-do' to think about. Cooking times will vary depending on how thick or thin you like your bases.

Ingredients

4 x 700 ml bottles passata (puréed tomatoes)

8 garlic cloves, crushed

4 teaspoons sugar

4 tablespoons olive oil

4 tablespoons fresh chopped or dried herbs, such as parsley and oregano

4 cups self-raising flour, plus extra for dusting

4 cups Greek yoghurt

4 cups grated cheese, such as mozzarella or cheddar

Method

1. Preheat the oven to 220°C.
2. Combine the passata, garlic, sugar, olive oil, herbs and 160 ml water in a large saucepan. Bring to the boil over a high heat. Careful, the sauce will start to splatter as it simmers. Reduce the heat to low–medium and simmer the sauce until it thickens and reduces by half. Remove from the heat and set aside to cool.
3. In a large bowl, combine the flour and Greek yoghurt and mix well to form a dough. Add a little more flour or yoghurt if you feel the dough is too wet or too dry.
4. Divide the dough into 4 even-sized balls. On a clean work surface dusted with flour, roll the balls to your desired pizza base size and thickness.
5. If you don't have a pizza stone, lightly grease two baking trays. Place 2 pizza bases on each tray. Par-bake the bases for 5–10 minutes until the bases are just firm to the touch. Or for a crisper pizza, continue cooking until the dough starts to colour. Remove from the oven and set aside to cool.

6. Top each base with the tomato sauce and sprinkle with cheese.
7. Wrap each pizza in a layer of plastic wrap and then a layer of foil to avoid freezer burn.

Serving Suggestion

If desired, add extra toppings to your frozen pizzas and cover with more cheese, before popping in the oven to finish cooking. Serve with a green salad.

Storage & Reheating

The pizzas can be frozen when par cooked. Cool completely, then wrap well in plastic wrap and foil. To cook from frozen, preheat the oven to 220°C and cook until golden.

Yakitori Chicken Kebabs

Makes approximately 30 x 16 cm-long kebabs

Easy to make in big batches and keep tucked away in the freezer, kebabs are MamaBake session favourites, the world over.

Ingredients

1 cup tamari or regular soy sauce

1 cup mirin

6 tablespoons honey

4 teaspoons ground ginger

8 garlic cloves, crushed

2 teaspoons sesame oil

1.5 kg chicken breasts or boneless chicken thighs, diced

Method

1. Soak the skewers in water while you prepare the ingredients.
2. Combine the soy sauce, mirin, honey, ground ginger, garlic and sesame oil in a large mixing jug.
3. Thread four pieces of chicken onto each skewer and set aside in a large baking dish. Pour over the marinade and give the kebabs a good wriggle until they are covered in the sauce. Pop on a lid or cover with plastic wrap and set aside in the fridge to marinate for a few hours or, preferably, overnight.

★ **At this point, you can either freeze all of the kebabs in their marinade or divide and put some in the freezer ready for defrosting and cooking another night.**

4. Heat a grill pan or frying pan over high heat and with a little marinade brushed over, grill or fry the kebabs in batches, until cooked through.

Serving Suggestion

This dish is perfect for a quick dinner served with sautéed kale or steamed broccoli. It is also wonderful with steamed rice and delicious wrapped in a flat bread or tortilla with lettuce.

Storage & Reheating

Prior to cooking, the kebabs can be frozen in their marinade in a few zip lock bags.

Oven-Baked Butter Beans with Vegetables

Serves approximately 4 families of 4

'Serves 4' doesn't feature in my mother-in-law's vocabulary and food is always prepared in vast quantities as if a celebration could take place at any moment. Family dinners see a table laden with food: rice and potatoes, salads and vegetables, meat and cheese … The list goes on. We always go home with at least two containers of leftovers, so dinner at Eleni's place is like a MamaBake without having to cook!

I love these beans. Served hot and sprinkled with chunks of good feta, it makes a perfect evening meal or lunch. You could mix up the vegetables according to what's in season and enjoy this dish year-round.

Ingredients

6 onions, chopped into thick chunks

6 red capsicums, thickly sliced

9 carrots, cut into thick chunks

6 celery stalks with leaves, thickly sliced

6 tomatoes, chopped

3 x 400 g tins whole peeled tomatoes

3 tablespoons sweet chilli sauce (use gluten free, if needed)

1½ cups olive oil

6 cups vegetable stock (use gluten free, if needed)

pinch of ground cumin

9 x 400 g tins butter beans, drained and rinsed

2 big bunches parsley, leaves and stems chopped

Method

1. Preheat the oven to 180°C.
2. Combine the onion, capsicum, carrot, celery and tomato in a large bowl. Divide the prepared vegetables among two large or three regular-sized roasting tins and spread evenly.

3. In a separate large bowl, combine the tinned tomatoes, sweet chilli sauce, olive oil, stock and cumin. Season with salt and pepper. Pour the stock mixture, as evenly as you can manage, over the vegetables (reserving some of the liquid if the tins look too full).
4. Cook, uncovered, for approximately 1 hour, or until the vegetables are cooked and the sauce has begun to thicken. Remove from the oven, divide the beans among the tins and stir.
5. Cover with foil and return to the oven for a further 20–30 minutes or until everything is cooked through and the sauce has thickened a little. Remove from the oven and stir through the parsley.
6. Serve hot or cold.

Serving Suggestion

This dish is gorgeous sprinkled with feta and eaten with chunks of crusty bread. It can also work as a side dish to grilled chicken or lamb.

Storage & Reheating

The cooked and cooled beans will keep for 3 days in the fridge. They can also be frozen, but omit the parsley and add when cooking.

Spinach & Ricotta Pancakes
(gluten free)

Serves approximately 4 familes of 4

This recipe is easily adapted to make as many pancakes as you need and they keep beautifully in the fridge for a few days. They make a great snack or an easy lunch when teamed with some salad.

Ingredients

2 tablespoons butter

2 tablespoons olive oil, plus extra for shallow-frying

115 g gluten-free self-raising flour

3 cups milk

4 eggs, lightly beaten

2 cups firmly packed shredded spinach or silverbeet leaves

4 tablespoons fresh dill, chopped

4 spring onions, chopped

500 g ricotta

Method

1. Melt the butter and 2 tablespoons oil in a large saucepan over low heat. Add the flour, stir and 'cook' for a minute or so.
2. Remove from the heat and slowly add the milk, stirring all the time. Add the eggs, while continuing to stir – the mixture should thicken to resemble pancake batter (see note).
3. Add the spinach or silverbeet, dill, shallot and ricotta and stir to combine.
4. Heat a little olive oil in a heavy-based frying pan and cook individually (a ladleful), as you would regular pancakes.

   Note: You are trying to achieve a béchamel-style thin white sauce. If the mixture doesn't thicken, pop it back on a low heat and stir constantly until it thickens slightly.

Serving Suggestion

These pancakes are fantastic served with beetroot dip or tzatziki, or just rolled up and eaten on their own.

Storage & Reheating

These pancakes are best kept refrigerated and consumed within 3 days. If you do freeze them, wrap very well in plastic wrap. To cook from frozen, defrost overnight in the fridge and heat in a warm pan or microwave, although the texture will soften on defrosting.

Pastitsio – Greek Pasta Bake
(gluten free)

Makes 4 medium-sized bakes (to serve 4–6) or
2 large bakes (to serve 8–10)

A firm MamaBake family favourite, this Greek version of lasagne is comfort food at its finest. If gluten is not an issue for you, simply replace the gluten-free pasta and flour with regular versions.

Ingredients

1 kg gluten-free penne
4 cups grated parmesan
olive oil

2 small onions, chopped
1 kg beef mince
1 x 800 g tin whole peeled
    tomatoes

White sauce

6 tablespoons butter
splash of olive oil

3 cups gluten-free plain flour
2 litres milk

Method

1. Preheat the oven to 180°C.
2. Cook the pasta in plenty of salted boiling water until al dente. Drain and place in a large bowl. Toss through 2 cups of the grated parmesan.
3. To make the white sauce, heat the butter and the olive oil in a large saucepan. Remove from the heat and gradually stir in the flour, mixing all the time.
4. Return to a low heat and stir for a minute or so. Slowly add the milk, whisking all the time. Bring to a simmer and stir until the sauce thickens. Add the remaining parmesan and season with salt and pepper. Remove from the heat and set aside.

5. Heat a little olive oil in a large frying pan. Add the onion and sauté, stirring frequently, until translucent. Add the mince and stir until well browned, about 5 minutes. Add the tomatoes and simmer for 25–30 minutes, or until the meat is cooked and the sauce is thick. Season, to taste.
6. Preheat the oven to 180°C.
7. To assemble the bakes, stir ⅔ cup of the white sauce into the cooked pasta and cheese. Add the mince mixture and stir through. Divide the pasta among four medium-sized baking dishes or two large, deep dishes and cover with the remaining sauce.
8. Cook, uncovered, for 25 minutes.
9. Remove from the oven and sprinkle over the remaining 2 cups of grated parmesan. Return to the oven and bake for a further 20 minutes or until the top is golden brown.

Serving Suggestion

Pastitsio is a hearty meal and is best served with a simple salad or steamed green vegetables.

Storage & Reheating

Once cooked and cooled, this dish can be frozen, well covered.

To cook from frozen, defrost overnight in the fridge then reheat in a warm oven or microwave until thoroughly heated through.

Rich Beef Stew with Parmesan Dumplings

Serves approximately 4 families of 4

Using budget cuts of meat, this nifty, thrifty stew turns into a decadent family meal after a spot of slow cooking and dressing up with delicious steamed parmesan dumplings.

Ingredients
Stew

2 tablespoons olive oil

4 pieces osso bucco (about 1–1.2 kg in total)

2 onions, finely chopped

8 celery stalks, finely diced

6 carrots, finely diced

6 garlic cloves, finely chopped

2 cups red wine

4 x 400 g tins whole peeled tomatoes

600 ml beef or chicken stock

10 rosemary sprigs, leaves picked

2 teaspoons salt

1 teaspoon black pepper

2 cups chopped parsley

Parmesan Dumplings

500 g plain flour, plus extra for dusting

2 teaspoons baking powder

1 teaspoon salt

1 cup grated parmesan

200 ml milk

240 g butter, cubed

Method

1. Preheat the oven to 150°C.
2. Heat the oil in a large casserole dish over medium heat. Add the osso bucco and brown on either side before removing and setting aside on a plate.
3. In the same dish over medium heat, add the onion, celery and carrot and sauté until the onion is translucent, about 8 minutes. Add the garlic and cook for a further few minutes but do not let it brown.

4. Return the meat to the dish and turn the heat to high. Add the red wine and simmer for 3–5 minutes to let the alcohol cook off. Add the tomatoes, stock, rosemary leaves and salt and pepper and stir to combine.
5. Pop the lid on the casserole dish and cook in the oven for 1½–2 hours or until the meat is falling away from the bones.
6. Meanwhile, pulse the ingredients for the dumplings in a food processor or blender. Alternatively, combine the flour, baking powder, salt and cheese in a large bowl. Rub the butter into the dry ingredients until it resembles rough breadcrumbs. Gradually add the milk and stir to form a loose dough. Flour your hands and form the dough into golf ball-sized dumplings.
7. Remove the stew from the oven and return to a medium heat on the stovetop.
8. Place the dumplings on the top of the stew and press lightly. Replace the lid and gently simmer for 15–20 minutes or until the dumplings are cooked through. Alternatively, bake the dumplings in the oven alongside the stew for about 10–15 minutes or until light golden. Garnish generously with the fresh chopped parsley.

Serving Suggestion

The addition of dumplings makes this a complete meal in itself; however, it teams beautifully with a side of sautéed mushrooms or simple steamed greens.

Storage & Reheating

The cooked and cooled stew will keep for up to 1 week in the fridge or 3 months in the freezer. Separate the dumplings and keep them in an airtight container to stop them from breaking down in the stew. You can make the dumpling dough up to 3 days in advance but do not cook them in the stew until the day you plan to eat them. To cook from frozen, defrost overnight in the fridge, then reheat the stew in a saucepan until it is at simmering point. Add the parmesan dumplings and continue cooking.

Roast Pumpkin Gnocchi

Serves approximately 2 families of 4

If, like us, your potato gnocchi attempts are more like wallpaper glue than delicious dumplings, give these pumpkin morsels a try!

Ingredients

1 small pumpkin, seeds removed and cut into large chunks

canola, sunflower or grapeseed oil, for drizzling

½ cup grated parmesan

3 eggs

freshly grated nutmeg

3 cups plain flour, plus extra for dusting

Method

1. Preheat the oven to 190°C.
2. Place the pumpkin on a baking tray and drizzle over a little oil and season with salt and pepper. Roast the pumpkin for 30 minutes, or until soft.
3. Scrape the pumpkin flesh from the skins and purée in a food processor or blender. Transfer to a large bowl and stir through the parmesan. Season, to taste. Add the eggs one at a time and beat to combine. Grate about half a nutmeg into the mixture.
4. Add the flour 1 cup at a time, mix through a little and then add the next cup. It helps to start this process using a big spoon and then finish by hand because it's really sticky. You might be tempted to add more flour at this point. Add no more than ½ cup extra; otherwise, the gnocchi will not be tender.
5. Scrape the dough onto a floured work surface and cut into 8 pieces. Roll each piece of dough into a long snake 2–3 cm thick. Don't worry about making it perfectly even. Cut the strips into gnocchi, about 2–3 cm long.

* **At this point, the gnocchi can be frozen. Place on a well-floured baking tray and freeze. Once frozen, transfer to zip lock bags and return to the freezer.**

6. Bring a large saucepan of salted water to the boil and add the gnocchi, about 20 at a time. When they float to the top, they're done – this will take about 3 minutes. Remove the gnocchi using a slotted spoon and transfer to a lightly oiled bowl. Repeat with the remaining gnocchi and serve with your favourite sauce.

Serving Suggestion

These gnocchi are beautiful served with a few strips of grilled bacon, spinach and minced garlic (1 clove) cooked in a little butter and a large handful of grated parmesan.

Storage & Reheating

Uncooked gnocchi can be frozen for up to 1 month and cooked from frozen, so you don't need to defrost.

Slow Cooker Apricot Chicken

Serves 4 families (approximately 16 serves)

A big-batch, slow cooker version of a retro classic.

Ingredients

2 tablespoons ground cumin

2 tablespoons ground coriander

2 teaspoons ground cinnamon

4 cm piece ginger, roughly chopped

8 garlic cloves, roughly chopped

4 tablespoons coriander stems

2 kg boneless chicken thighs, trimmed and each thigh cut in half

4 tablespoons honey

4 tablespoons lemon juice

2 x 850 ml tins apricot nectar

500 g dried apricots

cornflour

Method

1. Combine the cumin, coriander, cinnamon, ginger, garlic and coriander stems in a food processor and pulse to finely chop.
2. Place the chicken in a large bowl and coat with the spice mix. Set aside in the fridge to marinate while you prepare the sauce.
3. Whisk the honey and lemon juice into the apricot nectar.
4. Lay the chicken pieces in the slow cooker (7-litre capacity) and pour the sauce on top. Stir through the dried apricots and season with salt and pepper.
5. Cook on LOW for 8 hours. In the last hour of cooking, stir through a little cornflour and continue to cook with the lid off to thicken the sauce.

Serving Suggestion

This rich meal works well served hot over brown rice garnished with coriander leaves and slivered almonds.

Storage & Reheating

Once cooked and cooled, the apricot chicken can be frozen, well covered.

To cook from frozen, defrost overnight in the fridge then reheat thoroughly in a microwave or saucepan.

Tuna, Quinoa & Broccoli Burgers
(gluten free)

Makes approximately 24 burgers

Kids love these burgers and it's a great way to get some green vegetables into them! The trick to ensuring that these patties stay together during cooking is to make sure that the vegetables are really, really finely chopped.

Ingredients

1 cup quinoa
1 onion, finely chopped
4 garlic cloves, finely chopped
1 head broccoli, finely chopped
1 cup almond meal (substitute regular or gluten-free breadcrumbs for nut allergies)

6 eggs, lightly beaten
450 g tinned tuna
oil of your choice for frying

Method

1. Place the quinoa and 3 litres of water in a saucepan. Bring to the boil and simmer for 12 minutes. Drain and set aside to cool.
2. Process the onion, garlic and broccoli in a food processor until finely minced (the less chunky the mix, the better the patties will stick together). Alternatively, finely chop the ingredients by hand.
3. Transfer the broccoli and onion mixture to a large bowl and add the almond meal, eggs and cooked quinoa. Add the tuna, mix well and season with salt and pepper, to taste.
4. Form the mixture into palm-sized patties, and set aside in the fridge to set a little.

★   **At this point the patties can be frozen between layers of baking paper in an airtight container.**

5. Heat the oil in a heavy-based frying pan over low–medium heat and cook, in batches, for about 4 minutes each side (ensure that you flip the burgers carefully as these babies are a little on the fragile side!). Drain on a paper towel-lined chopping board or plate.

Serving Suggestion

These burgers are great in a bagel with iceberg lettuce and avocado. They also work well in burger buns with a tartare sauce, or even as a stand-alone meal with a side salad and dipping sauce.

Storage & Reheating

These burgers can be frozen, uncooked or cooked, once completely cooled. Reheat thoroughly in a frying pan or microwave. Defrost thoroughly before cooking.

Vegetarian Sausage Rolls

Makes 48 sausage rolls

This recipe is incredibly versatile, as you can add your choice of nuts and cheese. These sausage rolls are perfect for lunchboxes and a great energy sustainer for Mama about mid afternoon.

Ingredients

6 eggs

2 small onions, roughly chopped

2 cups grated cheese of your
   choice

1½ cups chopped nuts

4 tablespoons soy sauce

1½ cups finely grated carrot

1 cup breadcrumbs

2 cups rolled oats

6 sheets puff pastry

3 tablespoons milk

Method

1. Preheat the oven to 200°C.
2. Process the eggs, onion, cheese, nuts and soy sauce in a food processor until well combined. Transfer to a large bowl and mix in the carrot, breadcrumbs and rolled oats.
3. Cut the puff pastry sheets in half.
4. Spoon ¹⁄₁₂ of the mixture in the middle of each half sheet and form into a sausage shape. Roll up the pastry to enclose the filling. Cut each log into desired lengths and transfer to a baking tray. Brush with milk and prick with a fork.
5. Bake for 15–20 minutes until golden.

Serving Suggestion

Dunk in your favourite sauce! Or add a side salad for a simple, tasty, family meal.

Storage & Reheating

You can freeze the sausage rolls before you cook them or, alternatively, once they are cooked and cooled. Cook the sausage rolls from frozen on a baking tray in a 200°C oven until cooked through and golden brown.

Big Batch Breads

New York Bagels

Makes 16

Save yourself a small fortune by making your own New York bagels!

Ingredients

3 cups warm water

3 tablespoons granulated sugar

4 teaspoons dry active yeast

1 kg plain flour or high-gluten flour, plus extra for dusting and kneading

3 teaspoons salt

Method

1. Pour 1 cup warm water into a small bowl. Add the sugar and the yeast, but don't stir. Set aside for 5 minutes, then stir to dissolve the sugar and the yeast.
2. Combine the flour and salt in a large bowl. Make a well in the centre and pour in the sugar and yeast mixture. Pour 1¼ cups of the remaining warm water into the well. Begin to mix and continue adding the remaining warm water as you go. You want to create a firm dough.
3. Dust a clean work surface with flour and knead the dough for about 10 minutes. As you knead, work in as much of the surface flour as you can, creating a stiff dough. Put the kneaded dough back in the bowl and set aside, covered, in a draft-free space to rise for 1 hour, or until doubled in size.
4. After the dough has doubled, punch it down then set aside to rise again for a further 10 minutes.
5. Divide the dough into 16 equal-sized balls. With a flour-covered finger, make a hole in the middle of each ball. Wiggle your finger around to make the hole bigger, until the dough resembles a bagel. Repeat with the remaining dough.
6. Place the bagels on a lightly greased baking tray, cover with a tea towel and set aside to rest for a further 10 minutes.
7. Preheat the oven to 220°C.

8. Bring a large saucepan of water to the boil then reduce to a simmer. Working in batches, drop each bagel into the water and remove when it rises to the surface.
9. Transfer the bagels back to the baking tray and sprinkle over your choice of toppings (e.g., sesame seeds, caraway seeds, poppy seeds).
10. Bake in the oven for 20 minutes or until golden brown. Allow to cool a little on a wire rack.

Serving Suggestion

We can't go past these smothered in cream cheese and topped with smoked salmon and chives.

Storage & Reheating

The bagels can be frozen once cooked and cooled. Defrost on the kitchen bench or pop in the toaster or oven.

Cheesy-Mite Scrolls

(gluten free)

Makes 24 small scrolls

Packing a quick and easy gluten-free lunchbox can be difficult. More often than not, gluten-free breads don't make the tastiest sandwiches. Enter our gluten-free version of a much loved classic bakery treat!

Ingredients

1¾ cups milk (plus an extra ¼ cup if the mix is too dry)

2 tablespoons psyllium husks

4 cups gluten-free self-raising flour

2 tablespoons caster sugar

100 g softened butter, chopped

4 tablespoons good quality gluten-free yeast 'mite' spread

2½–3 cups grated tasty cheese

Method

1. Preheat the oven to 200°C. Grease a 20 cm x 30 cm baking tin.
2. Pour the milk into a bowl and stir in the psyllium husks. Set aside for 10 minutes.
3. Sift the flour and sugar into a large bowl. Rub the butter into the flour with your fingertips until the mixture resembles breadcrumbs.
4. Pour in the milk mixture and stir well to combine. Use your hands to finish the mixing – you want to have a soft, sticky dough. Divide the dough in half and knead one half for 1 minute.
5. Line your kitchen bench with plastic wrap or baking paper, then roll the dough out into a rectangle (or something that kind of resembles one!). Spread 2 tablespoons of the yeast spread onto the dough (I used my fingers to get it going then finished it with a knife). Try to avoid any thick clumps of spread. Cover with cheese as evenly as you can.
6. Carefully lift the long side of the pastry and roll, using the plastic wrap or baking paper to assist you, as you would a sushi mat. Trim the ends and cut into 3 cm slices. Place the scrolls, cut side up, in the prepared baking tin.

7. Repeat steps 5–6 with the remaining dough.
8. Bake in the oven for about 35 minutes or until cooked through. Serve warm.

Storage & Reheating

The scrolls can be frozen once cooked and cooled. Lay flat in a zip lock bag or airtight container. Defrost overnight in the fridge and pop them in a hot oven to crisp up again.

If not eating the scrolls straightaway, allow to cool then store wrapped in plastic wrap in an airtight container for up to 3 days.

English Muffins

Makes 36 muffins

Breakfast is looking stress-free with our big-batch English Muffins!

Ingredients

2½ cups milk

120 g butter

2 eggs

1 cup Greek or natural yoghurt

4 cups wholemeal flour

4 cups plain flour, plus extra
 for dusting

5 teaspoons dry active yeast

3 tablespoons sugar

3 teaspoons salt

handful cornmeal or polenta

Method

1. Warm the milk in a small saucepan. Add the butter and stir to melt, but don't let this mixture get too hot. Remove from the heat and set aside to cool. When the mixture is just warm, whisk in the 2 eggs and the yoghurt. Set aside.
2. Combine the flours, yeast, sugar and salt in a large mixing bowl. Slowly add the liquid mixture while stirring with a large wooden spoon or your hands. Alternatively, use a stand mixer with a dough hook attachment. Mix until thoroughly combined – the mixture should be quite wet.
3. Cover with plastic wrap and set aside to rise for 1–2 hours or until doubled in size.
4. Dust a clean work surface with a generous amount of flour and scrape the dough onto it. Dust the top of the dough with flour and, using your hands or very gently with a rolling pin, press or roll the dough out until it is evenly 2–3 cm thick.
5. Dust a ring mould with flour and cut out dough rounds. Use a wide egg flipper or spatula to lift them from the work surface and place on a baking tray dusted with flour. Cover and allow to rest and rise for 30 minutes.
6. Preheat oven to 180°C.

7. Heat two non-stick frying pans or skillets over medium heat. Dust the pans with cornmeal or polenta then place a few dough rounds in each pan (you should be able to fit 2–4 in each, with ample space between so it's not difficult to flip them).
8. Toast on each side for 3 minutes until golden brown. Place the toasted muffins on a baking tray lined with baking paper. When you have filled one tray, place it in the oven to finish cooking the muffins, about 8 minutes.
9. Tap the base of a muffin to hear if it makes a hollow sound. If it does, it's ready. If not, put them back in the oven for a further 1 minute then test again.

Storage & Reheating

Allow to cool before freezing the muffins in batches of however many you think your family will consume each morning. Pop them in the toaster unsliced for a minute or two to defrost, then slice in half and toast again.

Sesame & Chia Bread Rolls

(gluten free)

Makes 10–12 rolls

Finally! A gluten-free roll that has the texture of 'real' bread and can be eaten untoasted! These rolls are delicious – fluffy enough to be satisfying and 'bready', even on the second day, and freeze like a dream.

Ingredients

3 cups gluten-free self-raising flour

⅔ cup LSA

80 g psyllium husks

2 tablespoons chia seeds

3 tablespoons sesame seeds (plus extra for sprinkling)

2 tablespoons raw sugar or honey

pinch of salt

2 x 7 g sachets dry active yeast

650 ml warm water

2 eggs, lightly beaten

80 ml light oil (we use macadamia)

rice flour, for dusting

milk for brushing

sea salt, for sprinkling

Method

1. Grease a 20 cm x 30 cm baking tin.
2. Mix the flour, LSA, psyllium husks, seeds, sugar or honey and the salt in a large bowl.
3. In another bowl, dissolve the yeast into the warm water and set aside for a few minutes to activate – about 10 minutes.
4. Pour the yeast and water into the flour mixture and mix well. Add the beaten egg and oil and mix again – the dough should be wet and sticky. Cover and set aside to rise in a warm spot for around 30 minutes.
5. Generously dust a clean work surface with rice flour and tip out the dough. Using well-floured hands, gently fold the dough in on itself to form a ball. Stretch out the dough into a long sausage shape and divide into 10–12 rounds. Place the rounds in the baking tin and leave, uncovered, somewhere warm to rise again for 30 minutes.
6. Preheat the oven to 220°C.

7. Brush each dough round with a little milk and sprinkle with sea salt and some extra sesame seeds.
8. Bake for about 35 minutes or until the tops of the rolls are golden.

Serving Suggestion

There's nothing better than a still-hot roll from the oven, slathered in butter! Or fill them with your favourite lunchtime combination.

Storage & Reheating

These freeze beautifully after cooking and cooling.

Ham & Cheese Monkey Bread Rolls

Makes 16 rolls

Our savoury version of the cult bakery item, Monkey Bread!

Storage & Reheating

You can freeze the filled, prepared dough in a baking tin, covered in plastic wrap really tightly. When you want to bake it, unwrap the rolls and place in the oven as soon as you turn it on. As the oven warms, the bread will defrost and prove. Follow step 6 to cook.

Ingredients

550 g plain flour, plus extra for dusting

2 teaspoons dry active yeast

2 teaspoons salt

3 tablespoons oil

370 ml warm water

8 slices good quality ham, chopped

400 g cheddar or tasty cheese, grated

Method

1. If using a stand mixer, add the flour, yeast, salt and oil to the bowl and mix with dough hook attachment on the lowest setting, gradually adding the warm water. Knead for 8 minutes. If making the dough by hand, mix the ingredients in a large bowl until the dough comes together. Knead for at least 15–20 minutes on a well-floured clean surface until the dough is elastic and silky.
2. Transfer the dough to a large metal bowl greased with a little oil and cover with a clean tea towel. Set aside to rise until doubled in size – on a warm day this will take 1 hour; on a cold day 2–2½ hours.
3. Preheat the oven to 170°C and line an 18 x 18 cm baking tin with baking paper.
4. Once risen, scrape the dough onto a well-floured clean surface. Divide the dough into 16 equal-sized balls. Roll the dough balls or flatten with your palm until they are about 1.5 cm thick.

5. Fill each piece of dough with a little ham and cheese until you have used up all the filling. Pinch the edges of the dough around the filling and seal well. Place the filled dough balls in the prepared tin.

★ **You can freeze the dough at this stage.**

6. Bake for 30–40 minutes, or until the middle of a bread roll feels firm when pressed and the top is golden. Cool slightly before consuming because the cheese will be hot.

Big Batch Sweet Treats

Easy Honey Cake

Makes 2 x 20 cm round cakes

There's something about cakes made with honey that transports me back to my childhood. This is a simple, wholesome and delicious cake that kids and adults alike simply adore!

Ingredients

400 g unsalted butter, plus extra for greasing

500 g honey

160 g brown sugar

6 eggs

600 g self-raising flour

Method

1. Preheat the oven to 160°C. Grease and line two 20 cm round cake tins.
2. Place the butter, honey and sugar in a medium-sized saucepan over low heat. Bring to the boil, then remove from the heat and set aside to cool until just warm.
3. Transfer the mixture to a large mixing bowl, then add the eggs one by one and whisk thoroughly to combine. Gently fold in the flour, then pour the mixture into the prepared tins.
4. Bake each cake for 45–55 minutes or until the centre of the cake springs back when pressed and the top is a deep golden colour. Allow to cool before removing from the tins.

Serving Suggestion

This cake is lovely and dense, so lends itself well to being cut and sandwiched with jam and cream.

Storage

The cake will keep, well wrapped in plastic wrap in an airtight container, for up to 1 week in the fridge or 3 months in the freezer.

Baked Cinnamon Sugar Doughnuts

Makes 12–14 doughnuts and 12–14 doughnut holes

For a special treat every now and then, homemade doughnuts are simply delightful!

Ingredients

450 g plain flour

2 teaspoons instant dried yeast

55 g sugar

1 teaspoon ground cinnamon

pinch of salt

1 egg

1 cup milk

90 ml melted unsalted butter or oil

For coating

½ cup melted butter

170 g caster sugar

2 tablespoons ground cinnamon

Method

1. Place the flour, yeast, sugar, cinnamon and salt in a large mixing bowl or the bowl of a stand mixer. Whisk the egg and milk in a small bowl, then add to the dry ingredients. Mix well to combine.
2. If using a stand mixer, set the speed to low and gradually add the melted butter or oil. Alternatively, knead in the butter or oil by hand. Continue to knead the dough for 4–5 minutes, until it is smooth and elastic. Cover with plastic wrap and set aside to rise for 1 hour or until increased in size by about one-third.
3. Scrape the dough onto a lightly floured work surface and roll out to a 2 cm-thick circle. Using a large 8–10 cm round cutter, cut circles from the dough and transfer to a lined baking tray.
4. Using a small 2 cm round cutter, cut holes from the centres of the dough circles. Place these on a separate lined baking tray as they will take less time to bake.
5. Set the trays aside in a warm place and allow to rise, covered, for an additional 30 minutes.
6. Preheat the oven to 170°C.

7. Bake the doughnut rings for about 15 minutes or until light golden. Bake the doughnut holes for 8–10 minutes.
8. Meanwhile, melt the butter for the coating, then transfer to a small bowl. In a separate bowl, combine the sugar and cinnamon. Allow the doughnuts to cool a little, then brush each doughnut in butter before rolling in the cinnamon sugar. Repeat with the remaining doughnuts and serve.

Storage

The doughnuts will keep in an airtight container for 3–5 days or wrapped well in the freezer for 2–3 months.

Banana & Apple Loaf Cake

Makes 2 loaf cakes

A great recipe to use up those overripe bananas lurking in the fruit bowl. The riper the banana, the better the cake.

Ingredients

250 g softened unsalted butter, plus extra for greasing

360 g dark brown sugar, plus extra for sprinkling

700 g overripe bananas, mashed

2 teaspoons vanilla extract

2 teaspoons ground ginger or cinnamon

4 eggs

600 g plain flour

2 teaspoons baking powder

1½ teaspoons bicarbonate of soda

1 apple, cored and chopped into small chunks

Method

1. Preheat the oven to 180°C. Grease and line two loaf tins.
2. Using a stand mixer, beat together the butter and sugar until creamy and pale. Beat in the mashed bananas, then add the vanilla, ginger and eggs and mix to combine. Sift in the flour, baking powder and bicarbonate soda, then fold through the apple chunks.
3. Divide the batter between the loaf tins and sprinkle over a little extra brown sugar for a sweet caramel crunch, if desired.
4. Bake for about 1 hour, or until a skewer inserted into the middle of the cake comes out clean. Leave to cool in the tins for 5 minutes, then transfer to a wire rack to cool completely before slicing.

Storage

This cake freezes beautifully once cooled and cut into slices. Simply remove from the freezer in the morning and it will be ready to eat by morning tea time! This cake will keep for up to a week in an airtight container.

Sticky Date Puddings with Caramel Sauce

Makes 4 big puddings

This is a great sweet treat for a MamaBake session. Or, if you're MamaBaking solo, pop one on the table (your family will never forgive you if they all end up in the freezer!) and serve with cream or ice cream.

Ingredients

680 g dried dates, chopped

4 teaspoons bicarbonate of soda

240 g butter, softened

680 g brown sugar

8 eggs, lightly beaten

2 teaspoons vanilla extract

680 g self-raising flour

Caramel Sauce

800 g brown sugar

400 ml cream

500 g butter

Method

1. Preheat the oven to 150°C. Grease four 20 cm round cake tins.
2. Place the dates, bicarbonate of soda and 1 litre of water in a large saucepan and bring to the boil. Reduce the heat and cook until the dates start to break down.
3. Remove from the heat and transfer to a large heatproof bowl. Add the butter and stir through until fully combined. Add the sugar, egg and vanilla and stir to combine. Fold in the flour.
4. Divide the mixture evenly between the cake tins. Bake for about 1 hour, or until a skewer inserted into the centre of the puddings comes out clean.
5. Meanwhile, to make the caramel sauce, place the sugar, cream and butter in a saucepan and bring to the boil. Reduce the heat and simmer until golden brown. Allow the caramel sauce to cool, then divide among four containers to be served with the puddings when reheated.

Storage

The cooked and cooled puddings can be frozen for up to 6 months. The sauce should not be frozen but can be refrigerated for up to 3 days in the fridge (and is in fact the most delicious fudge-y sauce direct from the fridge). Defrost cakes overnight and reheat in microwave until heated through thoroughly. Cakes can be stored in the fridge for up to a week and can be reheated using the microwave or in a 180°C oven, covered.

Banana Slab Cake
(gluten free)

Serves 12–16

I don't know about you, but come 3 pm, a 'slab' of cake sounds just about perfect!

125 g softened unsalted butter, plus extra for greasing

220 g sugar

110 g coconut sugar or brown sugar

2 eggs

1 teaspoon vanilla extract

3–4 ripe bananas, mashed

300 g plain gluten-free flour (or substitute regular plain flour)

1 teaspoon baking powder

1 teaspoon ground cinnamon

125 g sour cream

½ teaspoon salt

Icing

180 g cream cheese

60 g very soft butter

250 g icing sugar

1 teaspoon vanilla extract

1 tablespoon lemon juice, to taste

Method

1. Preheat the oven to 180°C. Grease and line a 30 cm x 20 cm lamington tin.
2. Using a stand mixer, beat the butter and sugars until creamy and pale. Beat in the eggs, then mix in the vanilla and mashed banana. Add the flour, salt, baking powder, cinnamon and sour cream. Mix well.
3. Pour into the prepared tin and spread evenly.
4. Bake for about 20 minutes or until a skewer inserted into the middle of the cake comes out clean. Cool for 5 minutes in the tray, then invert onto a wire rack and set aside to cool completely.

★ **At this point, the cake can be frozen.**

5. To make the icing, beat all of the icing ingredients with an electric mixer until smooth and creamy. Pour over the cake and allow to set before slicing.

Storage

The cake will keep in an airtight container for up to 3 days in the fridge. The un-iced cake will keep for up to 1 month in the freezer, well wrapped. Defrost thoroughly before consuming.

Chocolate Chip & Raisin Biscuits

This recipe makes a BIG batch of BIG biscuits! You'll get a least
24 palm-sized biscuits from this mix, or more if you make them smaller.

Dense and just sweet enough, these are great for a quick and
nutritious grab-and-go breakfast on those mornings when getting out
the door fully clothed can be a struggle.

Ingredients

200 g instant oats
180 g almond flour
140 g sunflower seeds
130 g pumpkin seeds (pepitas)
80 g shredded coconut
170 g coconut sugar
1 teaspoon ground cinnamon
pinch of salt

240 g chopped dark chocolate
or chocolate chips
125 g raisins
70 g molasses
150 g coconut oil, melted
and cooled
240 ml coconut milk

Method

1. Preheat the oven to 180°C. Line two baking trays with baking paper.
2. In a large bowl, mix all of the dry ingredients until well combined,
   making sure to break up any lumps of coconut sugar. In a separate
   bowl, combine the molasses, coconut oil and coconut milk with
   ¼ cup water.
3. Pour the wet ingredients into the dry and mix until just combined.
   Fill a ⅓ measuring cup with the mix and transfer to one of the
   prepared trays. Flatten slightly with the back of a spoon, then repeat
   with the remaining mixture.
4. Bake for 25 minutes or until lightly golden, then set aside to cool on
   a wire rack.

Storage

These biscuits freeze well and can be frozen, well wrapped, for up to
2 months. They can be stored in an airtight container in the fridge for
up to 5 days. Defrost thoroughly before consuming.

Fudgy Cocoa Brownies

Makes 12–16, depending on brownie size

Craving brownies but there's no chocolate in the house? This is the 'emergency' brownie recipe every MamaBaker needs!

Ingredients

140 g unsalted butter, plus extra
    for greasing
220 g caster sugar
55 g brown sugar
½ teaspoon salt

1 teaspoon vanilla extract
90 g good quality cocoa powder
2 eggs
50 g plain flour

Method

1. Preheat the oven to 170°C. Grease and line a 25 cm x 25 cm baking tin.
2. Melt the butter in a medium-sized saucepan over low–medium heat until foaming and starting to brown. Remove from the heat and whisk in the caster sugar, brown sugar, salt, vanilla and cocoa powder, until the mixture looks thick and grainy. Set aside for 5–8 minutes to cool a little.
3. Add the eggs one at a time and whisk thoroughly to combine. The mixture will become smooth and silky. Gently fold through the flour, then scrape the mixture into the prepared tin and spread evenly with a spatula.
4. Bake for 20–30 minutes or until the centre is set and slightly puffed up. Cool completely before cutting into squares and serving.

Storage

The brownies will keep for up to 1 week in the fridge or up to 2 months in the freezer, wrapped well in plastic wrap, foil or in an airtight container.

Perfect Muffins

Makes 18 muffins

This is the no-fail muffin recipe you've been searching for.

Ingredients

300 g plain flour (or use a mix of plain white flour and wholemeal or alternative flours)

1 teaspoon baking powder

1 teaspoon bicarbonate of soda

pinch of salt

220 g sugar (or use a mixture of dark and light sugar, such as golden caster sugar and coconut sugar)

125 g butter, softened, plus extra for greasing

1 egg

1 cup buttermilk or plain yoghurt

2 cups filling of your choice (sweet or savoury)

Method

1. Preheat the oven to 190°C. Line a muffin tray with paper cases or grease 18 muffin holes. If you don't have muffin cases, you can also press squares of baking paper into the holes.
2. Combine the flour, baking powder, bicarbonate of soda and salt in a bowl.
3. In a separate bowl, cream together the sugar and butter until well combine. Add the egg, then beat in thoroughly, scraping the bottom of the bowl to ensure that there are no clumps.
4. Gently fold through the dry ingredients and buttermilk or yoghurt alternately. Finally, stir through your filling of choice. Don't over-mix.
5. Bake for 15–20 minutes until the muffins are golden brown and spring back when pressed in the centre.

Here are our tips for the perfect muffin fillings.

- Chop your fillings into small, bite-sized pieces. Larger chunks may not cook evenly or release too much moisture into the batter resulting in wet spots throughout the muffin.
- Fresh fruits such as apple, stone fruit, pear, berries and banana do not need to be pre-cooked before adding to the batter. You should only add 25 g of fruit; otherwise your muffins will be too wet.
- Dried fruit, seeds and nuts are great to mix into your muffins. Chocolate chips and coconut flakes are also delicious. Use your judgement if adding these ingredients, as you won't need as much as 2 cups.
- Add 1 teaspoon of sweet spices such as ground cinnamon.
- To make chocolate muffins, add 2 tablespoons of good quality cocoa powder.
- If you don't have buttermilk you can substitute natural yoghurt or make your own! Measure 1 scant cup of milk, then stir in 1 tablespoon of lemon juice or white vinegar. Set aside for 5–10 minutes at room temperature, then follow the instructions for using buttermilk in the recipe.

Storage

The muffins will keep, well wrapped, for 1 week in fridge and up to 1 month in the freezer.

Spicy Gingerbread Biscuits

Makes 30–40 biscuits

Perfect for Christmas time, and every month in between!

Ingredients

220 g softened butter

100 g brown sugar

60 g caster sugar

1 egg

170 g molasses (golden syrup or honey are fine, if you prefer a lighter gingerbread)

220 g wholemeal flour

300 g plain flour, plus extra for dusting

5 teaspoons ground ginger

3 teaspoons mixed spice

2 teaspoons ground cinnamon

1 tablespoon cocoa powder

1 teaspoon salt

Method

1. Using a stand or hand-held mixer, beat the butter and both sugars until pale and smooth. Add the egg and beat thoroughly to combine, then beat in the molasses until the mixture is evenly coloured.
2. In a separate bowl, combine the flours, spices, cocoa and salt. Gently fold this into the wet mixture to form a smooth dough.
3. Cut the dough into quarters, then wrap well in plastic wrap and set aside to chill in the fridge for at least 1 hour before rolling out.

* **At this point, the dough can be frozen.**

4. Preheat the oven to 160°C. Line a baking tray and set aside.
5. On a well-floured surface, roll out one piece of dough to about 1 cm thick. Cut the dough into 6 cm squares or cut 6 cm rounds using a cookie cutter.
6. Bake for about 8 minutes, or until the edges of the biscuits are lightly coloured but the centres are still soft. Transfer to a wire rack. The biscuits may seem soft, but they will firm up once cold.

Storage

The uncooked dough can be well wrapped and frozen for up to 2 months. Baked biscuits can be frozen, well wrapped, for up to 2 months.

Fruit Cake

Makes 5 x 1 kg cakes or 8 x 625 g cakes

It's never too early to start your Christmas baking!

Ingredients

1 kg sultanas

600 g currants

400 g raisins

300 g mixed peel

315 g marmalade

1 cup orange juice

1 cup brandy

1 cup port

440 g salted butter, plus
    extra for greasing

400 g brown sugar

8 eggs

600 g plain flour

4 teaspoons mixed spice

2 teaspoons ground cinnamon

2 teaspoons ground cardamom

1 teaspoon salt

Method

1. In a large bowl, combine the sultanas, currants, raisins, mixed peel, marmalade, orange juice, brandy and port. Set aside to soak for as long as possible for a minimum of one month (it will even last several months, if kept in the fridge).
2. Preheat the oven to 150°C. Grease and line the cake tins.
3. Using a stand or hand-held mixer, beat the butter and brown sugar until pale and fluffy. Whisk in the eggs one at a time until well combined. Add the flour, spices and salt and whisk thoroughly to combine. Stir through the dried fruit and the soaking liquid until well combined.
4. Divide the mixture among the cake tins (or cook one at a time if you don't have multiple tins of the right size). I use scales to ensure that each cake has the same amount of mixture.
5. Bake large cakes for 1–1¼ hours or small cakes for 30– 45 minutes or until a skewer comes out clean. Allow to cool completely before wrapping in plastic wrap and storing.

Storage

Fruit cake has a long shelf-life, so you probably won't need to freeze them. The cakes will keep, well wrapped, for up to 1 year in a cool, dark, dry place. To freeze, wrap well in plastic wrap, followed by foil, then freeze for up to 6 months. Allow 24 hours for the cakes to defrost.

Greek Honey Biscuits

Makes 40–50

These honey-rich, moist and crumbly biscuits are a must for a sweet treat at your next family celebration or MamaBake session.

Ingredients

250 g unsalted butter, softened
550 g caster sugar
3 eggs
1 cup vegetable oil
zest and juice of 1 orange
1 teaspoon vanilla extract
½ teaspoon ground cinnamon

½ cup red wine
1 teaspoon lemon juice
100 g walnut meal, plus extra
   for dusting
450 g self-raising flour, plus extra
   if necessary
250 g honey

Method

1. Preheat the oven to 160°C and line at least two baking trays with baking paper.
2. Using a stand or hand-held mixer, beat together the butter and sugar until pale. Add the eggs, one at a time, mixing well in between additions. Add the oil, orange zest and juice, vanilla, cinnamon, wine, lemon juice and walnut meal and mix on a low speed until combined.
3. Mixing by hand, gradually add the flour until the mix resembles a firm bread dough. Add a little more flour if your dough is still wet.
4. Form the dough into oval-shaped biscuits by gently rolling a heaped tablespoon of the mix in your hands. Place the biscuits on the prepared baking trays, then lightly press the tops with the back of a fork (don't flatten the dough).

★ **At this point, the uncooked biscuits can be frozen.**

5. Bake for 15 minutes, then remove from the oven and allow to cool completely.
6. Combine the honey with 1½ cups water in a medium-sized saucepan and bring to a gentle boil. Reduce the heat and simmer for 10 minutes. Set aside to cool a little.

7. Dip the biscuits into the melted honey, then dust with a little extra walnut meal.

Storage

Uncooked biscuits will keep, stored in an airtight container, for up to 4 months in the freezer. Cooked and uncoated biscuits can also be frozen for up to 2 months. Completed biscuits can be kept in airtight container in the fridge for up to a week.

Homemade Waffles

Makes 32 waffles

This is a basic recipe for sweet and savoury waffles. We've listed a few of our favourite fillings below, or feel free to make up your own.

Ingredients

600 g flour
2 teaspoons baking powder
1 teaspoon baking soda
2–4 tablespoons sugar
    (for sweet waffles)

4 cups milk
4 tablespoons white vinegar
1⅓ cups rice bran oil
4 large eggs
pinch of salt

Method

1. Combine the dry ingredients (including the sugar if making sweet waffles) in a large bowl and mix well. In a separate bowl, whisk together the milk, vinegar, oil and eggs.
2. Make a well in the dry ingredients and slowly pour in the wet ingredients, whisking as you pour. Whisk until the mixture is just combined and there are no lumps. Do not over-mix.
3. Heat your waffle iron, then fill each cavity three-quarters full with the waffle batter. Close the lid and cook according to the manufacturer's instructions.
4. Serve immediately with your choice of toppings.

Here are some of our favourite waffle fillings.

1. Ham, cheese and spring onion: add 80 g shredded ham, 125 g tasty cheese and 2 thinly sliced spring onions to the waffle batter.
2. Cornmeal and bacon: substitute 75 g flour with 75 g coarse polenta. Add 5 rashers of thinly sliced fried bacon.
3. Sweetcorn waffles: strip the kernels from 2 corn cobs and add to the waffle batter. Serve, topped with avocado and tomato.
4. Potato waffles: substitute 150 g flour with 230 g mashed potato.
5. Fruit waffles: add 130 g fresh fruit such as berries, diced stone fruit or chopped banana to the waffle batter.

6. Chocolate-chip waffles: add 90 g chocolate chips to your waffle batter. Particularly good with the addition of a chopped banana.
7. Cinnamon sugar waffles: add 2 teaspoons of ground cinnamon to a sweet waffle batter.

Storage

Leftover cooked waffles can be frozen and quickly reheated by popping them in the toaster. Waffles can also be stored in the fridge for a quick breakfast option.

Cooked waffles can be frozen for up to 1–2 months, fully wrapped. They will last up to one day in the fridge.

Classic Caramel Slice

Makes 1 large tray of slices

These are perfect for school fetes or a sneaky sweet treat with your afternoon cuppa!

Ingredients
Base

150 g flour

25 g rolled oats

50 g brown sugar

¼ teaspoon salt

60 g butter, chopped

1 egg

Caramel

200 ml condensed milk

55 g brown sugar

40 g butter

2 tablespoons golden syrup
(or use honey for a lovely
honey caramel)

Topping

80 g dark chocolate (70% cacao),
broken into pieces

¾ cup cream

Method

1. Preheat the oven to 175°C. Line the base of a 30 cm x 30 cm baking tin with baking paper.
2. For the base, combine the flour, rolled oats, brown sugar and salt in a large bowl. Add the butter and work into the dry ingredients until the mixture resembles breadcrumbs. Add the egg and work it in with your hands. Press the mixture into the prepared tin.
3. Bake in the oven for 15 minutes until light golden brown in the centre. Set aside to cool.
4. To make the caramel, combine the condensed milk, brown sugar, butter and golden syrup in a small saucepan over medium heat. Bring to the boil and stir constantly for 7 minutes, until the mixture is thick and pulls away from the side of the pan.
5. Pour the caramel over the cooled base, spread evenly and set aside.

6. To make the topping, place the chocolate in a small bowl. Bring the cream to a gentle boil in a small saucepan, then remove from the heat and pour over the chocolate. Whisk thoroughly to combine.
7. Spread the chocolate ganache over the caramel layer. Set aside in the fridge to set for 1 hour. Cut into 2–3 cm squares and serve.

Storage
The caramel slice will keep in the fridge for up to 1 week and should not be frozen.

Cookies & Cream Greek Yoghurt

Makes approximately 1.25 kg or serves 5 people

Admit it, who hasn't sat down at the end of a long day with a tub of Cookies & Cream ice cream and a spoon and eaten the whole thing?

Ingredients

1 kg Greek yoghurt
5 tablespoons almond butter
150 g chocolate chips

2½ teaspoons natural vanilla extract

Method

1. Empty the Greek yoghurt into a large bowl and stir through the almond butter. Add the chocolate chips and mix well, then add the vanilla extract and mix well to combine.
2. Divide among single-serve containers and set aside in the fridge or freezer.

Storage

The yoghurt can be frozen in single serve (1 cup) portions. To eat from frozen (ice cream anyone?), simply allow to defrost on the kitchen bench for 15 minutes to soften slightly.

This will keep in the fridge for up to 5–7 days or up to 1 month in the freezer.

Honey & Pear Muffins

(gluten & dairy free)

Makes 24 muffins

Comforting muffins – lovely for morning teas, perfect for lunchboxes, and minus the gluten and dairy.

Ingredients

600 g gluten-free plain flour

220 g coconut sugar, plus extra for sprinkling

1½ tablespoons gluten-free baking powder

pinch of salt

1 tablespoon ground cinnamon, plus extra for sprinkling

500 g coconut yoghurt

½ cup coconut oil

½ cup honey

2 eggs

2 teaspoons vanilla extract

4 pears, peeled, cored and diced

Method

1. Preheat the oven to 180°C. Line two 12-hole muffin tins with paper cases.
2. Combine the dry ingredients in a large bowl and mix well. In a separate bowl, combine the remaining ingredients except the pear and mix well.
3. Gently fold the wet ingredients into the flour mixture until just mixed through. Do not over-mix. Fold through the pear.
4. Using an ice-cream scoop or spoon, scoop the batter into the lined muffin tins, sprinkle with some extra coconut sugar and cinnamon and bake for 20–30 minutes. Serve warm.

Storage

The muffins can be placed in zip lock bags and frozen.

Defrost overnight in the fridge and warm through in a microwave or oven before eating.

These muffins can be kept in the fridge for 1 week and frozen for up to 2–3 months (well wrapped).

Honey Tart

Makes 2 tarts

A beautiful, rustic tart that just begs to be eaten on a tartan picnic rug while reading Enid Blyton. Alternatively, serve warm into hungry little hands for afternoon tea straight after school or reheat after dinner and serve with cream for an extra delicious factor.

Ingredients
Pastry
340 g plain flour, plus extra for dusting

pinch of sea salt

170 g cold butter, cubed, plus extra for greasing

Filling
½ cup honey

50 g fresh breadcrumbs

zest of 1 lemon or orange

2 tablespoons lemon or orange juice

Method
1. Preheat the oven to 200°C. Lightly grease two 23 cm tart tins.
2. Sift the flour and salt together in a large mixing bowl. Rub the butter into the flour using your fingertips until the mixture resembles fine breadcrumbs. Sprinkle up to 160 ml water onto the flour mixture, then stir together with a fork until you have a rough dough.
3. Turn the dough out onto a well-floured work surface and knead for a few minutes until you have a nice smooth dough. Wrap the dough in plastic wrap and pop to one side while you make the filling.
4. Heat the honey in a small saucepan over low heat until it becomes runny. Stir in the breadcrumbs, citrus zest and juice. Remove from the heat and set aside.
5. Divide the dough in half. On a lightly floured work surface, roll out one half to a circle slightly larger than your tart tin. Line the tin with the dough, then trim off any excess pastry and set aside. Repeat with the remaining half of dough.

6. Pour the filling into the pastry cases and spread evenly.
7. Roll out any leftover dough and cut thick strips to make a lattice topping. Alternatively, ask your kids to get creative!
8. Bake for 20–25 minutes, or until the pastry edges are lovely and golden brown.

Storage

The tarts will keep for up to 3 days in the fridge. They are not suitable for freezing.

Lamingtons

Makes 32 lamingtons

Our take on the classic Australian sponge cake. Rich with coconut, these take afternoon tea to the next level.

Ingredients

270 g desiccated coconut
160 ml boiling water
6 eggs
250 g caster sugar

50 ml canola, sunflower
or grapeseed oil, plus extra
for greasing
450 g self-raising flour

Coating

540 g desiccated coconut

Icing

875 g icing sugar
250 g cocoa powder

40 g melted butter
1½ cups milk

Method

1. Preheat the oven to 170°C. Grease and line two lamington tins.
2. Combine the desiccated coconut and just-boiled water in a medium-sized heatproof bowl. Set aside for 5 minutes for the coconut to rehydrate.
3. Place the eggs and sugar in the bowl of a stand mixer or large bowl, and whisk until pale and thick. Working in 6 batches, whisk in the oil, moistened coconut mixture and then the flour. Divide the mixture between the prepared trays.
4. Bake for 40–50 minutes or until the cake is golden brown on top and springs back in the centre when pressed. Remove from the oven and turn out onto wire racks to cool.
5. To make the topping, spread the desiccated coconut onto a large baking tray and toast in the residual oven heat for 3–5 minutes. Remove from the heat and transfer to a medium-sized bowl.

6. To make the icing, sift the icing sugar and cocoa powder into a large bowl and whisk to combine. Beat in the melted butter followed by the milk. Set aside.

7. When the cakes are cool, cut each cake into 16 squares. Using a fork, gently dip each cake square into the icing and ensure that all sides are covered before rolling in the toasted coconut. Place the coated squares on a lined baking tray and repeat with the remaining cakes.

8. Any leftover icing can be stored in the fridge for up to 1 week.

Storage

The lamingtons will keep for up to 1 week in an airtight container and are suitable for freezing. They will keep for up to 1 month in the freezer.

Lemon & Raspberry Cake

(gluten, grain & dairy free)

Makes 2 cakes

This is a lovely, rich, lemon-flavoured cake that is wonderful for MamaBakers who need to consider allergies.

Ingredients

oil, for greasing
100 g coconut flour
300 g almond flour
330 g sugar
½ teaspoon salt
3 teaspoons baking powder

6 eggs
zest of 2 lemons
2 tablespoons lemon juice
3 teaspoons vanilla extract
250 g frozen raspberries

Method

1. Preheat the oven to 190°C. Grease and line two loaf tins.
2. Combine the flours, sugar, salt and baking powder in a large bowl and mix well, making sure there are no lumps. In a separate bowl, lightly whisk the eggs, lemon zest and juice, vanilla and ½ cup water.
3. Pour the wet ingredients into the flour mixture and combine well until you have a smooth batter. Gently fold in the frozen raspberries, then pour into the prepared tins and smooth the tops with a spatula.
4. Bake for 35–40 minutes, or until a skewer inserted into the centre comes out clean. Turn the cakes out onto a wire rack to cool completely before slicing.

Storage

This cake is best kept in a container in the fridge and consumed within a few days. If you would like to freeze one of the cakes, wrap well in two layers of plastic wrap, then foil. Defrost overnight in the fridge to avoid it going mushy.

Granola Bars

(gluten free)

Makes 24 bars

A no-bake, melt-and-mix recipe for crispy granola bars. Use store-bought or homemade granola, or substitute all of the ingredients separately to tailor the bars to your own tastes. If replacing the granola with your own ingredients, ensure that two-thirds of the mix consists of oats and/or puffed rice, then add your other flavours to make up the remaining weight.

If you want to make these bars nut-free for lunchboxes, omit any nuts from the granola mix and use a sunflower seed butter instead of the nut butter.

Ingredients

700 g store-bought or homemade granola (or a mix of oats, puffed rice, nuts, seeds, berries etc.)

1 cup rice syrup

125 g nut butter

2 teaspoons vanilla extract

pinch of salt

Method

1. Line two 20 cm x 20 cm loaf tins with baking paper, ensuring that the paper comes up over the sides.
2. Place the granola or your own mix of ingredients in a large bowl.
3. Combine the syrup and nut butter in a medium-sized saucepan and gently heat until melted and combined. Add the vanilla and salt and stir through.
4. Pour the liquid into the granola and mix until thoroughly combined – this will take substantial elbow grease! Press the mixture into the prepared loaf tins and place in the freezer for a few hours until set.
5. Slice into 24 bars and enjoy!

Storage

These bars keep their crunch best if stored in an airtight container in the freezer for up to one month, but they can also be stored in the fridge for up to 2 weeks.

Honey Oat Bars

Makes 24 bars

These simple, honey-rich bars beg to be eaten with a good cup of tea!

Ingredients

4 tablespoons honey

220 g butter

220 g soft brown sugar

440 g rolled oats

1 teaspoon salt

2 teaspoons ground cinnamon

Method

1. Preheat the oven to 180°C. Line two lamington tins with baking paper.
2. In a medium-sized saucepan, melt the honey, butter and sugar over low heat, stirring occasionally. Remove from the heat, then add the remaining ingredients and stir well to combine.
3. Pour into the prepared tins and bake for 20 minutes. Allow to cool before cutting into 24 bars.

Storage

The bars will keep, stored in an airtight container in the fridge, for up to 1 week.

They can also be frozen, well wrapped in an airtight container, for up to 1 month.

Lemon, Ricotta & Almond Cakes

Makes 12 small cakes + 1 loaf

A beautiful recipe for a MamaBake session, particularly when lemons are in abundance!

Ingredients

500 g almond meal

2 teaspoons baking powder (use a gluten-free version, if required)

310 g caster sugar

500 g ricotta

4 eggs, beaten

zest of 6 lemons

180 g butter, melted, plus extra for greasing

Method

1. Preheat oven to 180°C. Grease and line a loaf tin and grease a 12-hole muffin tray.
2. Combine the almond meal, baking powder and sugar in a large bowl. In a separate bowl, combine the ricotta, beaten egg and lemon zest.
3. Add the wet ingredients to the almond meal mixture and fold through, gradually adding the melted butter as you go.
4. Pour the batter into the prepared loaf tin and muffin holes.
5. Bake the muffin cakes for 30 minutes and the loaf cake for 1 hour, or until a skewer inserted into the centre of the cake comes out clean.

Storage

These can be stored in the fridge for up to 1 week in an airtight container.

Honey Nut Brittle

Makes 2 sheets (enough for 4 families)

Rich with honey and full of crunch from the nuts, this is a much loved, classic confectionary that makes the perfect gift, or as a sweet, after-dinner treat for the family.

Ingredients

320 g butter

1 cup honey

280 g chopped nuts (substitute pumpkin seeds for a nut-free version)

Method

1. Line two baking trays with baking paper.
2. Place the butter and honey in a heavy-based saucepan over a medium–high heat and bring to the boil, stirring constantly. Heat the mixture to 300°C, using a sugar thermometer to assist you. This will take around 10 minutes and will be very, VERY hot! If you don't have a sugar thermometer, place a bowl of cold water next to the stovetop. Drizzle a little of the honey and butter mixture into the cold water. If the mixture hardens immediately, you have reached the 'hard crack' stage and the liquid is ready. If the mixture remains a liquid, then cook for a little longer and try again.
3. Stir in the nuts, then very carefully pour the hot mixture onto the prepared baking trays.
4. Set aside in the fridge until completely cold, then break into shards and store.

Storage

Keep this brittle in an airtight container in a cool, dark position. It is recommended not to store it in fridge or freezer.

Mini Chocolate Cupcakes with Chocolate Butter Icing

Makes 20 cupcakes

Perfect for children's birthday parties and a wonderful way to get kids involved in cooking.

Ingredients

450 g self-raising flour
60 g cocoa powder
230 g caster sugar
2 teaspoons vanilla extract

½ cup milk
160 g butter, softened, plus extra
   for greasing
4 eggs

Chocolate butter icing

100 g butter, softened
250 g icing sugar, sifted

40 g cocoa powder, sifted
2 tablespoons milk

Method

1. Preheat oven to 160°C. Grease two 12-hole muffin tins or line with cupcake cases.
2. Sift the flour and the cocoa powder into a large bowl. Add the sugar and mix to combine. Add the vanilla, milk, butter and eggs and mix until combined and glossy.
3. Pour into the prepared muffin tins and bake for 20 minutes. Remove from the oven and set aside to cool completely before icing the cakes.

★ **At this point, the un-iced cupcakes can be frozen.**

4. To make the icing, beat the butter in a stand mixer or with a hand-held mixer until pale and fluffy. Add the icing sugar and cocoa a little at a time until fully incorporated. Add the milk and mix until light and fluffy.
5. Spread onto the completely cooled cupcakes and serve.

Storage

Allow to cool completely before chilling or freezing. The un-iced cupcakes will keep for 1–2 days in the pantry, up to 7 days, well wrapped in the fridge or up to 4–6 months, well wrapped, in the freezer.

Portuguese Custard Tarts

Makes 12 tarts

Who doesn't love a Portuguese custard tart?

Ingredients

400 g (about 3 sheets) puff pastry
110 g sugar
1 cinnamon stick
1 tablespoon plain flour

¾ cup milk
¼ teaspoon vanilla extract
4 egg yolks

Method

1. Preheat the oven to 220°C.
2. If your pastry is in a block, roll it out to 2 mm thick. Cut out circles using an 8–9 cm biscuit cutter. Press each circle gently into a greased 12-hole muffin tin and set aside.
3. Combine the sugar, cinnamon and ⅓ cup water in a small saucepan and, using a sugar thermometer to assist you, cook until the liquid reaches 100°C. Remove from the heat and set aside to cool slightly.
4. In a large bowl, whisk the flour and ¼ cup milk. Set aside.
5. In another saucepan, add the remaining milk and the vanilla and bring to a simmer. Remove from the heat, then immediately whisk this mixture into the flour and milk.
6. Remove the cinnamon stick from the sugar syrup, then pour the syrup into the milk mixture in a thin stream, whisking the whole time. Whisk in the egg yolks quickly and thoroughly.
7. Fill each puff pastry shell three-quarters full with the custard mixture.
8. Bake for 8–10 minutes, until the pastry is golden and the custard has dark spots. Remove from the oven and allow to cool to just warm before serving.

Storage

These tarts will keep, stored in an airtight container in the fridge, for up to 3 days. The tarts should not be frozen. Reheat in a 160°C oven until warm.

Raspberry, Mango & Almond Slice
(gluten & grain free)

Makes 2 slices

Perfect for making the most of mango season, this slice is moist and sweetened naturally with fruit. It makes a lovely morning or afternoon tea in the summer months and is delicious warm, straight out of the oven, with a dollop of cream or ice cream.

Ingredients

4 mangoes, flesh roughly mashed

6 eggs separated

140 g sugar

500 g almond meal

2 teaspoons ground cinnamon

1 teaspoon baking powder

500 g frozen raspberries

Method

1. Preheat the oven to 180°C. Line two 26 cm x 16 cm slice tins.
2. Place the mango, egg yolks and sugar in the bowl of a stand mixer or large bowl and whisk until frothy. Add the almond meal, cinnamon and baking powder and mix until combined.
3. In a separate bowl whisk the egg whites until stiff peaks form. Carefully fold the egg whites into the cake batter, then fold in the frozen raspberries.
4. Pour the mixture evenly between the tins and bake for 40 minutes until golden on top or until a skewer inserted into the centre of cakes comes out clean. Allow to cool for 5 minutes in the tin, then remove and set aside on a wire rack to cool completely.

Storage

The cakes will keep, well wrapped in plastic wrap, for up to 1 week in the fridge and up to 3 months in the freezer.

Homemade Pink Marshmallows

Makes: the final quantity will depend on how big you cut your marshmallows, but you should have enough for about 3 families

Soft, pillowy marshmallows minus all the colourings and additives! These are perfect with hot chocolate, roasted over an open fire or for a sweet afternoon treat.

Ingredients

½ cup strawberry purée (hull whole strawberries, purée in blender or food processor and strain through a sieve) from approximately 1 punnet of strawberries

440 g caster sugar
2 tablespoons powdered gelatine
½ teaspoon vanilla extract
60 g icing sugar

Method

1. Line a 30 cm x 20 cm lamington tin with baking paper.
2. Place the strawberry purée into a small saucepan. Add the caster sugar and place over a low–medium heat.
3. In a small bowl, mix the gelatine in ½ cup water and set aside for at least 5 minutes.
4. Bring the strawberry and sugar mixture to the boil, then stir in the gelatine mix and vanilla until well combined. Boil for 1 minute, then remove from the heat.
5. Pour the mixture into the bowl of a stand mixer or a large metal bowl. Whisk on high speed, or use a hand-held mixer, for 3–5 minutes until tripled in size. When soft peaks form, scrape the marshmallow into the prepared tin and spread evenly.
6. Allow to set at room temperature for at least 2 hours. (Do not cover and do not place in the fridge. At this stage the marshmallow is both setting and drying, and any moisture trapped inside by refrigeration or covering will cause the marshmallow to 'weep'.)

7. Once set, dust the top of the marshmallow with 1 tablespoon of the icing sugar before turning out onto a chopping board. Slowly peel the paper from the marshmallow. If it is set, the paper will peel off and the marshmallow will bounce back into shape. Dust the rest of the marshmallow with a little icing sugar, then cut into shapes before dusting with the remaining sugar.

Storage

Marshmallows are unsuitable for freezing, but they will keep in an airtight container in a cool, dry place for up to 3 months.

Lime Macaroons
(gluten free)

Makes 32

One bowl. Four ingredients. Mix. Bake. Devour.

Ingredients
360 g desiccated coconut

230 g sugar

4 egg whites

3 tablespoons lime zest

Method
1. Preheat the oven to 180°C. Line two baking trays with baking paper.
2. Place all of the ingredients in a large bowl and mix well. Shape into walnut-sized balls and transfer to the baking trays.
3. Bake for 12–17 minutes or until the tops are lightly golden. Transfer to a wire rack to cool completely.

Storage
Allow to cool completely before chilling or freezing. Wrap the macaroons, in batches, in plastic wrap, then place in an airtight container. They will keep for up to 6 months in the freezer. Allow to defrost at room temperature. These macaroons can be stored for up to 2 days in the fridge.

Vanilla Blondies

Makes two 20 cm x 20 cm tins

Meet the 'Blondie', the delicious caramel sister to the much loved Brownie.

Ingredients

240 g butter, diced
450 g brown sugar
2 eggs
2 teaspoons vanilla extract
1 teaspoon salt

250 g plain flour
2 cups filling (chocolate chips, toasted nuts, coconut flakes, candy-coated chocolates, dried fruit, pretzels)

Method

1. Preheat the oven to 180°C. Line two 20 cm x 20 cm lamington tins with baking paper.
2. Place the butter in a heatproof bowl and transfer to the oven while it heats up. When the butter is slightly melted remove from the oven. Add the brown sugar and beat until smooth and starting to pale. Beat in the eggs one at a time until thoroughly combined. Add the vanilla and salt and beat to combine. Fold through the flour and stir until combined. Do not overmix.
3. Stir through your choice of filling, then divide the batter between the two tins.
4. Bake for 20–25 minutes, until golden on top and the centre is no longer runny. Allow to cool for at least 10 minutes before slicing into squares.

Storage

The blondies will keep, in an airtight container in the fridge, for up to 10 days. The blondies will also keep, well wrapped in plastic wrap, for up to 3 months in the freezer.

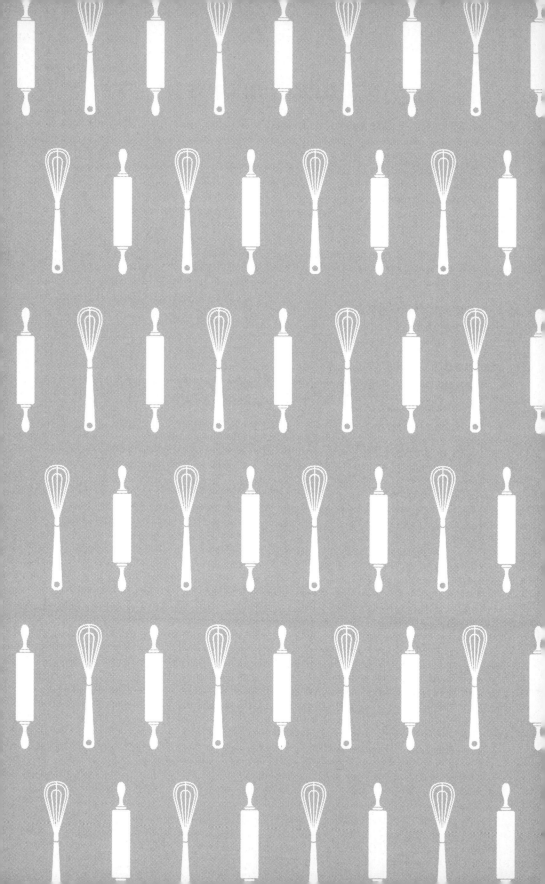

Big Batch Sauces,
Marinades,
Dips & Jams

Tomato Paste Two Ways

Makes approximately 2 cups

It's something we don't think twice about purchasing from the supermarket, but you can make your own tomato paste simply and easily at home, and know exactly what is going in it. If you like, experiment by adding different dried herbs for pizza bases.

1. Fresh Tomato Paste

½ cup olive oil, plus 4 tablespoons
4 kg ripe red tomatoes, roughly
   chopped

2 teaspoons salt

Method

1. Preheat the oven to 150°C. Grease a large baking dish with the 4 tablespoons of oil.
2. Heat the oil in a large stockpot over high heat. Add the tomatoes and bring to the boil. Cook, stirring frequently, for 10 minutes or until the tomatoes have softened.
3. If you would like a smooth paste, press the mixture through a sieve or food mill into a small bowl, to remove the seeds.
4. Spread the tomato mixture in the baking dish. Bake for about 3 hours, turning the tomatoes with a spatula every 20–30 minutes to evaporate the water.
5. Reduce the heat to 110°C and cook for a further 30 minutes, until the paste is thick and dark red.

Storage

Allow to cool completely before chilling or freezing. The tomato paste will keep in a sterilised glass jar in the fridge for 1 month, or stored in zip lock bags in the freezer for 6–8 months.

2. Quick Tomato Paste

3 x 400 g tins whole peeled or
    crushed tomatoes

80 ml olive oil
2 teaspoons salt

Method

1. Purée the tomatoes in a blender or food processor.
2. Place the puréed tomato, olive oil and salt to a medium-sized saucepan and bring to the boil over medium–high heat. Cook, stirring frequently, for 10–12 minutes or until the sauce has reduced by one-third.

Storage

Allow to cool completely before chilling or freezing. The tomato paste will keep in a sterilised glass jar in the fridge for 1 month, or stored in zip lock bags in the freezer for 6–8 months.

Teriyaki Sauce

Makes approximately 4 cups
(allow ½ cup marinade per 500 g ingredients)

Teriyaki sauce is super useful to have in your fridge for the upcoming week. You can put it on almost anything – meat, fish, tofu, any kind of vegetable – and transform a meal!

We love our homemade teriyaki sauce because we know what is going into it – the bottled stuff from the shops can have all sorts of unknowns in it, and it can be expensive.

This recipe is really quick and easy to make and only needs 3 ingredients.

Ingredients

½ cup soy sauce

½ cup mirin

2 tablespoons sugar or honey

3 cm piece piece ginger (optional)

Method

1. Place the soy sauce, mirin and up to 2 tablespoons sugar or honey (depending on how sweet you like your teriyaki sauce) in a small saucepan. Bring to a simmer and stir to dissolve the sugar or honey.
2. Simmer for about five minutes, stirring frequently. The sauce should reduce to a sticky but pourable consistency. The longer you cook it, the thicker and stickier the sauce will be.

Storage

If you are preparing meals for the week ahead, simply place the cooled teriyaki sauce and ingredients of your choice in a zip lock bag, then shake to ensure that the ingredients are well coated. Set aside in the freezer.

Defrost overnight in the fridge, then follow individual recipe instructions to cook.

Homemade Tomato Sauce

Makes approximately 4 cups

This recipe is fantastic to have in the fridge throughout a busy week. It is incredibly versatile and can be used as a base for many different meals such as pasta, pizza and meatballs. It's a lot healthier than the store-bought versions and, of course, much cheaper.

Ingredients

2 x 700 ml bottles of passata
4 garlic cloves, minced
2 bunches basil

2 tablespoons sugar
2 tablespoons olive oil
4 tablespoons of water

Method

1. Place all of the ingredients and ⅓ cup water in a heavy-based saucepan over high heat.
2. Once the mixture starts to splutter, reduce the heat to medium and cook, stirring occasionally, for about 20 minutes, until the sauce has reduced and thickened.

Storage

You can use the sauce straightaway on pizza and pasta.

Allow to cool completely before chilling or freezing. The tomato sauce will keep in a sterilised glass jar in the fridge for 1 month, or stored in zip lock bags in the freezer for 9 months.

Morello Cherry Balsamic Marinade

Makes approximately 2½ cups
(allow ½ cup marinade per 500 g meat)

A fruity, sweet marinade that goes beautifully with chicken.

Ingredients

1 cup balsamic vinegar

1 cup Morello cherry jam

1 cup olive oil

2 tablespoons minced garlic

2 tablespoons dried oregano

2 tablespoons cracked black
pepper

Method

Place all of the ingredients in a large bowl and whisk to combine.

Storage

This marinade will keep in a sterilised glass jar in the fridge for up to
1 week, or stored in zip lock bags in the freezer for up to 1 year.

If you are preparing meals for the week ahead, simply place the
marinade and meat of your choice in a zip lock bag, then shake to
ensure that the ingredients are well coated. Set aside in the freezer.

Defrost overnight in the fridge, then follow individual recipe
instructions to cook.

Mild Coconut Curry Simmer Sauce

**Makes approximately 7 cups
(enough for two family-sized curries)**

This is a very tasty, yet mild curry sauce. It's fantastically versatile and useful to have in the fridge for the week ahead.

Add diced chicken and vegetables, or meatballs. Prawns are particularly delicious added with some Asian greens and served with rice.

Ingredients

80 ml coconut oil

4 teaspoons finely minced ginger

2 teaspoons finely minced fresh or ground turmeric (optional)

4 garlic cloves, finely minced

2 tablespoons curry powder

2 teaspoons garam masala

2 x 400 g tins diced tomatoes

2 x 400 g tins coconut cream

1 teaspoon salt

1 teaspoon ground black pepper

Method

1. Melt the coconut oil in a heavy-based saucepan over medium heat. Add the ginger and turmeric (if using fresh) and cook for 1 minute. Add the garlic and stir for a few seconds. Add the curry powder, garam masala and turmeric (if using ground), and stir until fragrant. Add the tomatoes, coconut cream, salt and pepper and stir to combine.
2. Bring to the boil, then simmer, stirring occasionally, for approximately 20 minutes until thickened. If you are using the sauce straightaway, continue cooking and follow individual recipe instructions.

Storage

Allow to completely cool before chilling or freezing. The sauce will keep in a sterilised glass jar in the fridge for up to 5 days.

Lemongrass & Coconut Marinade

Makes approximately 2 cups
(allow ½ cup marinade per 500 g meat)

This is a delicately flavoured, delicious marinade for chicken and fish.

Ingredients

1 cup coconut oil, melted

1 cup rice wine vinegar

12 cloves garlic, finely minced

6 cm piece ginger, finely chopped

80 ml tamari

4 lemongrass stalks, bruised

Method

Place all of the ingredients except the lemongrass in a large bowl and whisk to combine. Add the lemongrass after whisking and remove when meat has finished marinating.

Storage & Reheating

This marinade will keep in a sterilised glass jar in the fridge for up to 1 week, or stored in zip lock bags in the freezer for up to 1 year.

If you are preparing meals for the week ahead, simply place the marinade and meat of your choice in a zip lock bag, then shake to ensure that the ingredients are well coated. Set aside in the freezer.

Defrost overnight in the fridge, then follow individual recipe instructions to cook.

Honey, Soy & Orange Marinade

Makes approximately 2½ cups
(allow ½ cup marinade per 500 g meat)

This is a classic marinade loved by families everywhere. We've added orange for a twist and extra flavour.

Ingredients

juice of 1½ oranges
1 cup soy sauce
1 cup runny honey
½ cup light olive oil

2 teaspoons finely minced ginger
1 teaspoon finely minced garlic
zest of 1 orange

Method

Place all of the ingredients in a large bowl and whisk to combine.

Storage

This marinade will keep in a sterilised glass jar in the fridge for up to 1 week. This recipe is unsuitable for freezing.

If you are preparing meals for the week ahead, simply place the marinade and meat of your choice in a zip lock bag, then shake to ensure that the ingredients are well coated. Set aside in the freezer.

Defrost overnight in the fridge, then follow individual recipe instructions to cook.

Fava

Makes approximately 4 cups

How do I explain Fava? It looks like hummus, but tastes nothing like it. It's part dip, part spread, part light, standalone meal. It's delicious on bread or as a warm dip for vegetables.

We love it with loads of lemon juice, salt and a spring onion chopped and stirred through, then warmed and eaten straight from the bowl.

You can also garnish and stir through any flavourings that take your fancy.

Ingredients

440 g yellow split peas 1¼ onions, grated

Method

1. Place the split peas and 1 grated onion in a large stockpot and fill with water. Bring to the boil and simmer, covered, for 2 hours over low heat. Do not lift the lid and do not stir!
2. Once the peas are soft and disintegrating, pour the mix, in batches, into a blender or food processor and blend with the remaining ¼ grated onion until smooth.
3. Fava is best served warmed. Once chilled, it will firm up quite quickly, so give it some gentle heat and a good stir before serving.

Serving Suggestion

Serve with spring onions sprinkled over the top, a drizzle of lemon juice and oil and crusty bread or flatbreads for dipping.

Storage

Allow to completely cool before chilling. Fava will keep for up to 1 week in the fridge. This recipe is unsuitable for freezing.

Dijon, Lemon & Oregano Marinade

Makes approximately 2½ cups
(allow ½ cup marinade per 500 g ingredients)

This is a tangy and light marinade that works particularly well with chicken. It is also delicious with barbecued vegetables.

Ingredients

1 cup lemon juice

1 cup olive oil

2 tablespoons dried oregano

190 g Dijon mustard

2 teaspoons minced garlic

Method

Place all of the ingredients in a large bowl and whisk to combine.

Storage

This marinade will keep in a sterilised glass jar in the fridge for up to 1 week, or stored in zip lock bags in the freezer for up to 1 year.

If you are preparing meals for the week ahead, simply place the marinade and meat or vegetables of your choice in a zip lock bag, then shake to ensure that the ingredients are well coated. Set aside in the freezer.

Defrost overnight in the fridge, then follow individual recipe instructions to cook.

Homemade Barbecue Sauce

Makes approximately 4 cups

This lovely, spicy sauce made with whole-food ingredients is a total winner on the family dinner table. It can be served with all the usual suspects – sausages, burgers and steaks – but it is also a knock-out on vegetables such as roasted whole sweet potatoes stuffed with barbecued kidney beans and avocado.

Ingredients

2 teaspoons olive oil
2 red onions, finely chopped
2 garlic cloves, minced
1 teaspoon smoked paprika
1 teaspoon mustard powder
2 teaspoons chilli powder
    (optional)

2 x 400 g tins crushed tomatoes
½ cup maple syrup
⅓ cup apple cider vinegar
2 tablespoons tamari

Method

1. Heat the oil in a medium-sized saucepan over medium heat. Add the onion and garlic and gently cook, stirring, for about 3 minutes. Add the smoked paprika, mustard powder and chilli power (if using), and stir to coat the onion and garlic. Add the tomatoes, vinegar, maple syrup and tamari and stir to combine.
2. Bring to a gentle boil, then reduce the heat and simmer for about 10 minutes or until thickened.

Storage

Allow to cool completely before chilling. The barbecue sauce will keep stored in a sterilised glass jar in the fridge for 2–3 weeks.

Lemon Curd

Makes approximately 3 cups

This is a *delicious* recipe that can be used in so many ways. We find that the most popular method of consumption is to scoop spoonfuls directly out of the jar and into one's mouth. Gosh, it's *that* good.

Great for little lemon tarts, on Greek yoghurt or ice cream, or slathered on toast or scones.

Ingredients

3 eggs, well beaten

240 g caster sugar

zest and juice of 2 lemons

120 g butter, cut into small cubes

Method

1. Fill a saucepan with water and place over a low heat. Place a heatproof bowl on top, making sure that the bowl isn't touching the water. Add the egg, sugar and lemon zest and juice to the bowl, then, whisking constantly, add the cubes of butter one at a time. Keep whisking until the lemon butter becomes thick and smooth.
2. Pass the butter through a fine-meshed sieve to make it even more smooth, if desired.
3. Pour your lemon curd into sterilised jars.

Storage

Allow to cool completely before chilling. The lemon curd will keep in a sterilised glass jar in the fridge for up to 3 weeks.

Homemade Raspberry Chia Jam

Makes approximately 4 cups

You can use fresh or defrosted frozen berries for this very simple and quick jam recipe.

Ingredients

500 g fresh or defrosted frozen raspberries

8 tablespoons chia seeds

juice of 2 lemons

2–4 tablespoons liquid sweetener such as honey, maple syrup, agave, rice bran syrup or stevia (optional)

Method

1. Mash raspberries with a potato masher or fork in a large bowl. Stir in the chia seeds and lemon juice. Add your choice of sweetener, to taste (if using)
2. Cover and set aside in the fridge for at least 1 hour.

Storage

The jam will keep stored in a sterilised glass jar in the fridge for up to 2 weeks.

Big Batch Homemade Packet Mixes

Big Batch Homemade Packet Mixes

Be they a helpful pantry-ready shortcut or a great gift for someone you know, dry-mix recipes can be really handy to have around.

Make-your-own packet mixes are easy to knock together and can be made in bulk for much less cost than the boxes and packs you can buy at the supermarket.

Most dry mixes will just need the addition of wet ingredients to turn them into something delicious.

Put together several dry-mix recipes on a MamaBake day and keep them in large, airtight containers or glass jars. These can keep for a month and, depending on the conditions they are stored in, much longer (depending on moisture levels where jars are stored).

Each of these mixes with the exception of the cake mix have a relatively long shelf life if kept in a well-sealed glass jar in a dark, cool cupboard.

We recommend that the cake mix is stored in the freezer due to the dairy ingredients.

Hot Chocolate Mix

Ingredients

4 cups milk powder
1½ cups icing sugar
2 cups good-quality cocoa powder

2 cups finely chopped milk or dark chocolate
1 teaspoon salt

How to use

Combine 1 tablespoon of the mix with 1 mug of hot water.

Malt Drink Mix

Ingredients

4 cups milk powder
1 cup malt powder

¾ cup cocoa powder

How to use

Combine 1 tablespoon of the mix with 1 mug of hot water or hot milk.

Pancake Mix

Ingredients

1 kg plain flour
5 tablespoons baking powder
3 teaspoons baking soda

¾ cup sugar
4 teaspoons salt

How to use

Add 1 egg and 1 cup of milk for every 1 cup of the mix. This mixture makes about 2–3 dozen pancakes, depending on their size.

Chocolate-Chip Cookie Mix

Ingredients

6 cups plain flour
1½ cups rolled oats
2 cups brown sugar
4 cups caster sugar

2 teaspoons baking soda
2 teaspoons salt
2 cups chocolate chips

How to use

Combine 4 cups of this mixture with 120 g butter and 1 egg, lightly beaten. Roll into tablespoon-sized balls, place on a lined baking tray and bake at 170°C for 15 minutes.

Cornbread Mix

Ingredients

6 cups plain flour

6 cups coarse or fine polenta

3 cups milk powder

7 tablespoons baking powder

5 teaspoons salt

How to use

Combine 2 cups of this mix with ½ cup butter, 2 eggs and ¾ cup of water. Pour into a lined loaf tin and bake for 15–20 minutes at 200°C.

Vanilla Cake Mix

This one is a little different, as you keep the mix in the freezer because it includes the fat component, which makes it even easier to throw together when you want to bake a cake.

Ingredients

6 cups plain flour

4 cups sugar

1 cup milk powder

2 tablespoons baking powder

3 teaspoons salt

3 teaspoons vanilla essence

2 cups chilled diced butter

How to use

1. Pulse the ingredients in a food processor and divide between two zip lock bags and freeze.
2. To make a cake, combine one bag of mixture with 2 eggs and 1¼ cups of water. Pour into a greased and lined cake tin and bake at 170°C for 20–30 minutes, or until the cake bounces back when pressed gently in the centre.

Cocoa Brownie Mix

Ingredients

1½ cups plus 1 tablespoon
  plain flour

1½ cups plus 1 tablespoon
  caster sugar

1½ cups plus 1 tablespoon
  brown sugar

1 cup plus 1 tablespoon
  cocoa powder

1 teaspoon baking powder

1 teaspoon salt

How to use

Combine 2 eggs and ½ cup of vegetable oil for every 2 cups of mixture.
Add 1 teaspoon of vanilla essence. Whisk together, pour into a greased
and lined 25 cm x 25 cm (or equivalent) baking tin and bake at 175°C
for 20–25 minutes. This mix should yield 3 batches of brownies.

Dry Soup Mix

Ingredients

2 cups yellow split peas

2 cups red lentils

2 cups green split peas

5 teaspoons chicken or vegetable
  stock granules

2 tablespoons sweet paprika

4 tablespoons dehydrated onion
  or onion powder

3 teaspoons garlic powder

2 teaspoons celery seeds

2 teaspoons dried parsley

2 teaspoons dried thyme

3 teaspoons salt

How to use

Combine 3 cups of this mixture with at least 2 cups of boiling water.
Allow to soak for 1 hour before bringing to the boil. This makes a basic
soup, but you can add fresh vegetables or dried pasta when you cook it.

Taco Seasoning

Ingredients

¼ cup ground cumin

¼ cup smoked paprika

½ cup chilli powder

½ cup onion powder

3 tablespoons garlic powder

2 tablespoons sea salt

How to use

Add 2 tablespoons to every 500 g of minced or diced meat.

Gravy Mix

Ingredients

2 cups plain flour

4 tablespoons meat-based
bouillon granules

1 teaspoon pepper

How to use

Melt 20 g of butter in a small saucepan. Stir through 2 tablespoons
of gravy mix and allow to bubble and brown slightly. Whisk in
¾ cup of water until smooth and allow to bubble for 2–3 minutes.

Index

Thank you

Deep gratitude and love to my husband, Denis, and my son, Alex, for their unwavering belief and support during the creation of this book. To my Mum, Bev Swan, for holding down the fort and making sure we were all taken care of as I hid away in the spare room with the laptop for days on end. Your love and support are priceless to me.

To my soul-sister Hannah Ireland for being as excited as I am about this project, for endless cups of tea, laughter and keeping up the chocolate supplies, I can't thank you enough.

And to Michelle, there's no-one else I'd rather be on this ride with than you!

– Karen

My heartfelt thanks to my husband, Steve, and our beautiful children, Mia and Alby, who supported me through the long hours of this book adventure. Love you all.

Also, to my beloved family in the UK and Australia for their encouragement.

And, of course, my thanks and gratitude to Karen for being an incredible friend and MamaBake partner for the past five-odd years. What a trip!

– Michelle

Karen and Michelle offer their abundant gratitude to the unique MamaBake community – thank you for your vibrancy, honesty, good humour, longstanding loyalty and support. We appreciate every one of you.

We also thank Emma Chow, who brought her amazing chef expertise and skills to the MamaBake table and made our Once-A-Week Cooking idea come to life. Thank you Emma, for your hard work and incredible dedication.

We would like to offer a huge thank you to Brigitta Doyle, Publishing Director of ABC Books and publisher of this book, who first spotted us and saw something in MamaBake that could be a book. Thanks for believing in us and for all your support in turning *The MamaBake Book* into a reality.

We are grateful to Jacinta di Mase, our agent, whose outstanding expertise has guided us through this first-time experience so smoothly. You have been a pleasure to work with and we thank you for leading us and for your unending support.

Our thanks to Barbara McClenahan, our editor, who has worked tirelessly with us, often burning the candle at both ends, to get this book to the finish line. Thank you for your eagle-eye and dedication to improving this book. Also, thank you Rachel Denis, who worked with us as our editor at the beginning of this process and did an extraordinary job of making sense of our hundreds of recipes and the cooking plans! Thanks, Rachel.

We thank also Lucy Heaver, who did an excellent job of trawling through the plans and recipes, tightening everything up. Thanks Lucy, that job wasn't for the faint-hearted and it looks terrific as a result of your work.

Also, to Hazel Lam, who did a beautiful job with the book design – we absolutely love it!

Michelle Shearer and Karen Swan are mothers who were united in their passion to free up women from the unending pressures of domestic burden through the power of The Sisterhood. They could see that by cooking together in one big hit just once a week they could share the workload with others and, even if going at it alone, big batch cooking afforded time off later in the week for mums everywhere.

Karen joined Michelle in the running of the MamaBake community a year after it was founded, in 2010, and together they have grown the family of MamaBakers to many thousands of women, as well as facilitated hundreds of real-life MamaBake groups across the world.

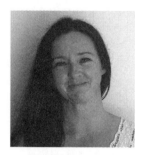

Michelle lives on the North Coast of NSW with her husband, two children and too many chickens, parrots and guinea pigs; grows her own food wherever possible; and is passionate about women's rights and the power of women as a collective.

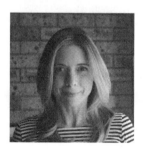

Karen lives in Canberra ACT with her husband and young son, and is passionate about helping women/mothers find the support, friendship and help they need to fully enjoy motherhood and continue to develop into the women they aspire to be. Karen appears regularly on ABC Radio to discuss all things food and women.

You can join the vibrant and friendly MamaBake community.
On Facebook: facebook.com/mamabakeHQ
At their website: mamabake.com
On Instagram: mamabakeofficial #mamabake